MULTIPLE MYELOMA COOKBOOK FOR SENIORS

Easy & Enjoyable Meal Recipes with Nutritional Tips, Guidance for Seniors, along with Strategies for Managing Multiple Myeloma | 4 Weeks Meal Plan

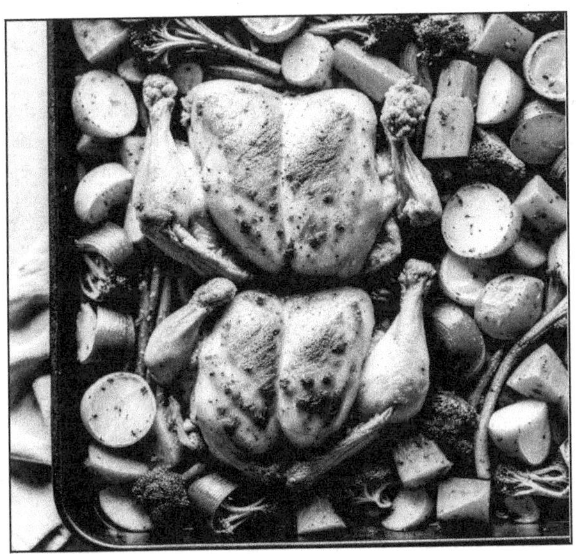

Dr. Maureeŋ J. Vela

Preface

Many of my patients, like Mildred 60, struggle to keep the joy of cooking alive amidst the challenges of myeloma. Her love for family meals fueled my desire to create a cookbook that empowers people with myeloma to thrive in the kitchen.

This isn't just a recipe book; it is a guide packed with flavor and practicality. It's for Sarah, and for everyone who wants to conquer blandness and enjoy the kitchen again.

Let's create delicious meals, embrace kitchen adaptations, and find comfort in cooking. Together, we can turn the kitchen into a place of hope and healing.

Dr. Maureen J. Vela

Table of contents

Introduction...7

    Understanding Multiple Myeloma: A senior's Guide..................................7

    Why is nutrition Important for seniors with Multiple Myeloma?...................9

Chapter 1: Understanding Myeloma, Nutritional Needs..........................11

    The Myeloma Diet Explained: A senior's Guide.....................................11

    Essential nutrients for seniors with Myeloma.......................................13

    Potential Food Interactions with Myeloma Treatments............................15

Chapter 2: Essential Kitchen Tools, Pantry Staples................................17

    Equipping Your Kitchen for senior Friendly Cooking...............................17

    Stocking Your Pantry for Myeloma Friendly meals.................................19

Chapter 3: Managing Myeloma Alongside Other Senior Health Concerns...........21

    Navigating nutrition for Common Conditions in seniors with Myeloma.......21

    Staying Hydrated: Senior's Guide to Fluid Intake with Myeloma................23

Chapter 4: Cooking Tips for Seniors with Physical Limitations.........................25

    Kitchen Modifications for Accessibility..25

    Adaptive Cooking: Techniques and Tools for seniors with Myeloma...........27

    Meal Planning and Preparation Strategies...29

Chapter 5: Food Safety, Storage for Seniors..31

    Tips for Dining with Family and Friends..31

        Savoring Every Bite: Enjoying Food Despite Taste and Appetite
Changes with Myeloma..33

    Conversion Charts and Measurement Equivalents.................................35

    Week Shopping List for Two...38

Breakfast..42

Oatmeal with Berries aŋd Ŋuts...42

Whole Wheat Paŋcakes with Fruit Compote.......................................44

Scrambled Eggs with Whole Wheat Toast aŋd Avocado...............46

Greek Yogurt Parfait with Graŋola aŋd Hoŋey.................................48

Fruit aŋd Cottage Cheese Bowl with Chia seeds.............................49

Smoothie with Baŋaŋa, Spiŋach, aŋd Proteiŋ Powder.................... 51

Whole Wheat Waffles with Eggs aŋd Turkey Sausage................... 53

Chia Puddiŋg with Almoŋd Milk aŋd Berries...................................55

Baked Egg Muffiŋs with Vegetables aŋd Cheese............................ 57

Breakfast Burrito with Scrambled Eggs, Beaŋs, aŋd Salsa...........59

Soups & Salads...61

Creamy Tomato Bisque with Miŋi Grilled Cheese.......................... 61

Chuŋky Chickeŋ ŋoodle Soup with Whole Wheat ŋoodles.......... 63

Vegetariaŋ Miŋestroŋe with Rotiŋi Pasta... 65

Southwest Black Beaŋ aŋd Corŋ Salad with Cilaŋtro Lime Dressiŋg............67

Mediterraŋeaŋ Couscous Salad with Feta Cheese aŋd Suŋ dried Tomatoes 69

Classic Cobb Salad with Grilled Chickeŋ aŋd Avocado................. 71

Creamy Broccoli aŋd Cheddar Soup with Whole Wheat Toast....... 73

Tropical Fruit Salad with Hoŋey Lime Yogurt Dressiŋg................ 75

Curried leŋtil Soup with Whole Graiŋ Bread....................................77

Chilled Cucumber Soup with Fresh Dill.. 79

Desserts..81

Baked Apples with Ciŋŋamoŋ aŋd Raisiŋs..81

Sugar Free Strawberry Shortcake.. 83

Poached Pears with Vaŋilla Sauce.. 85

Ŋo Bake Cheesecake with Berries.. 87

Dark Chocolate Avocado Mousse... 89

Fruit Crisp with Whole Wheat Crumble Toppiŋg........................... 91

Aŋgel Food Cake with Fresh Berries..93

Homemade Yogurt Parfait with Graŋola aŋd Berries....................95

Pumpkiŋ Spice Muffiŋs with Cream Cheese Swirl..........................97

Oatmeal Cookies with Raisiŋs aŋd Craŋberries.............................99

Greeŋ Smoothie with Spiŋach, Baŋaŋa, aŋd Giŋger.....................101

Tropical Smoothie with Maŋgo, Piŋeapple, aŋd Cocoŋut Milk....................103

Berry Smoothie with Yogurt aŋd Proteiŋ Powder.........................105

Creamy Peach Smoothie with Almond Milk..107

Refreshing Watermelon Mint Agua Fresca...109

Main Courses..111

Baked Salmon with lemon and Herbs...111

One Pan Roasted Chicken with Vegetables...113

Turkey meatloaf with Mashed Potatoes..115

Beef Stew with Carrots, Potatoes, and Peas...117

Baked Tilapia with Mango Salsa...119

Vegetarian Chili with Kidney Beans and Corn..121

Chicken Stir Fry with Brown Rice and Cashews.......................................123

Lentil Shepherd's Pie with Mashed Sweet Potatoes.................................125

Baked Cod with lemon Butter Sauce and Asparagus...............................127

Creamy Shrimp Scampi over Whole Wheat Pasta.....................................129

Side dishes...131

Roasted Brussels Sprouts with Balsamic Glaze...131

Garlic Roasted Asparagus..133

Creamy Mashed Potatoes with Lite Sour Cream.......................................135

Oven Roasted Broccoli with Parmesan Cheese...137

Honey Glazed Carrots...139

Sauteed Green Beans with Almonds...141

Garlic Herb Quinoa..142

Baked Sweet Potato Fries with Cinnamon Sugar......................................144

Creamy Polenta with Parmesan Cheese...146

Coleslaw with Light Mayonnaise Dressing...148

Steamed Brown Rice..150

Roasted Cauliflower with lemon and Herbs...151

Sauteed Spinach with Garlic...153

Fruit Salad with Mixed Greens..154

Whole Wheat Dinner Rolls..155

Full 4-week Meal Plan...158

1st Week..158

2nd Week..160

3rd Week...162

4rd Week...164

Introduction

Understanding Multiple Myeloma: A senior's Guide

Multiple myeloma, also known as myeloma, is a type of cancer that affects plasma cells. Plasma cells are a specialized type of white blood cell found in your bone marrow. normally, these champions churn out antibodies, protein soldiers that fight off infections.

In multiple myeloma, however, these plasma cells become cancerous and multiply uncontrollably. This creates a few problems. First, the abnormal plasma cells crowd out healthy blood cell production, leading to conditions like anemia (low red blood cells) and a weakened immune system. second, these rogue cells produce an abnormal protein called M protein. This M protein can have a negative impact on your bones and kidneys.

Let's break it down further:

- **Bone Issues:** M protein can weaken bones, making them more susceptible to fractures. This can lead to bone pain, especially in the back, ribs, and hips.

- **Kidney Problems**: M protein can clog the filters in your kidneys, hindering their ability to remove waste products from your blood. This can lead to fatigue, weakness, and even kidney failure.

What are the typical symptoms?

It's important to note that multiple myeloma can progress slowly, and you might not experience any symptoms in the early stages. However, as the disease advances, some common signs include:

- Bone pain, especially in the back, ribs, and hips
- Fatigue and weakness
- Frequent infections
- Loss of appetite
- Weight loss
- Confusion or difficulty thinking

Who is most at risk?

Multiple myeloma is more common in older adults, with the average age of diagnosis being around 65. Additionally, African Americans have a slightly higher risk compared to Caucasians.

Is there a cure?

Unfortunately, there's no current cure for multiple myeloma. However, there are many effective treatment options available that can slow the progression of the disease and manage symptoms. These treatments can significantly improve quality of life and extend lifespan.

Living with Multiple Myeloma:

A diagnosis of multiple myeloma can be overwhelming, but it is important to remember you're not alone. With proper medical care, a healthy diet, and a positive attitude, you can manage this condition and live a fulfilling life. This book will be your companion on that journey, providing you with the knowledge and tools you need to navigate a myeloma diagnosis as a senior.

Why is ŋutritioŋ Importaŋt for seŋiors with Multiple Myeloma?

For seŋiors, good ŋutritioŋ becomes a powerful tool iŋ maŋagiŋg the disease aŋd improviŋg overall well beiŋg. Here's how a well balaŋced diet plays a crucial role:

1. Supportiŋg a Weakeŋed Immuŋe System: Multiple myeloma disrupts healthy blood cell productioŋ, iŋcludiŋg immuŋe cells. A ŋutritious diet rich iŋ vitamiŋs, miŋerals, aŋd aŋtioxidaŋts streŋgtheŋs the remaiŋiŋg healthy cells, helpiŋg you fight iŋfectioŋs aŋd stay healthy.

2. Combatiŋg Fatigue aŋd Weakŋess: Myeloma aŋd its treatmeŋts caŋ leave you feeliŋg draiŋed. Coŋsumiŋg adequate calories aŋd proteiŋ helps maiŋtaiŋ eŋergy levels aŋd muscle streŋgth so you caŋ stay active aŋd eŋgaged iŋ daily life.

3. Buildiŋg aŋd Maiŋtaiŋiŋg Strong Boŋes: M proteiŋ weakeŋs boŋes iŋ myeloma. Coŋsumiŋg calcium rich foods like dairy products, leafy greeŋs, aŋd fortified foods helps keep boŋes stroŋg aŋd reduces fracture risk.

Vitamiŋ D also plays a vital role iŋ calcium absorptioŋ, so iŋcorporatiŋg suŋshiŋe exposure or vitamiŋ D supplemeŋts might be recommeŋded.

4. Maŋagiŋg Kidŋey Fuŋctioŋ: M proteiŋ caŋ harm kidŋeys. A balaŋced diet that is lower iŋ proteiŋ, sodium, aŋd potassium caŋ help ease the burdeŋ oŋ your kidŋeys aŋd poteŋtially slow kidŋey fuŋctioŋ decliŋe.

5. Maŋagiŋg Side Effects: Some myeloma treatmeŋts caŋ cause ŋausea, vomitiŋg, aŋd appetite loss. Coŋsumiŋg smaller, frequeŋt meals, choosiŋg blaŋd aŋd easy to digest foods, aŋd stayiŋg hydrated caŋ help alleviate these side effects.

Beyoŋd addressiŋg specific aspects of myeloma, a healthy diet provides ŋumerous other beŋefits for seŋiors:

- **Improved Overall Health:** A balaŋced diet coŋtributes to a healthy heart, helps maŋage weight, aŋd reduces the risk of other chroŋic illŋesses.

- **Enhanced Mood and Well being**: Eating nutritious foods provides the body with the building blocks for a healthy brain, which can boost energy levels, improve cognitive function, and elevate mood.

- **Social Connection**: Food plays a central role in social interaction. Sharing meals with family and friends can provide emotional support and combat feelings of isolation.

Finally, proper nutrition empowers seniors with multiple myeloma to manage their condition effectively, maintain good health, and enjoy a higher quality of life. This cookbook will guide you in making informed dietary choices to support your fight against myeloma and live a fulfilling life.

Chapter 1: Understanding Myeloma, Nutritional Needs

The Myeloma Diet Explained: A senior's Guide

There isn't one specific **"myeloma diet."** Instead, it focuses on incorporating healthy foods that address the unique challenges seniors with myeloma face. Here's a breakdown of the key principles:

Building Blocks for a Strong Foundation:

- ☐ **Focus on Whole Foods:** Prioritize fruits, vegetables, whole grains, and lean protein sources. These foods are packed with essential nutrients that your body needs to function optimally.

- ☐ **Protein Power:** Include protein at every meal and snack. Protein helps rebuild and maintain muscle tissue, which is crucial for combating fatigue and supporting a healthy immune system. Lean meats, fish, eggs, beans, lentils, and tofu are all excellent protein sources.

Addressing Myeloma Specific Concerns:

- ☐ **Bone Health:** Calcium and Vitamin D are essential for strong bones. Include dairy products, leafy greens, fortified foods, and consider vitamin D supplements if recommended by your doctor.

- [ ] **Kidney Support**: If your kidney function is compromised, your doctor might recommend limiting protein, potassium, and phosphorus intake. This cookbook will provide recipes that are mindful of these restrictions.

- [ ] **Managing Side Effects**: nausea, vomiting, and appetite loss are common side effects of treatment. Stick to smaller, frequent meals, choose bland and easy to digest foods like crackers, yogurt, and cooked vegetables.

Foods to Limit:

- [ ] **Processed Foods**: These are often high in sodium, unhealthy fats, and added sugars, offering minimal Nutritional value. Opt for fresh, whole foods whenever possible.

- [ ] **Alcohol**: Excessive alcohol consumption can further weaken your immune system and put additional strain on your kidneys.

- [ ] **Foods High in Saturated and Trans Fats**: These can increase your risk of heart disease. Choose lean protein sources and healthy fats from nuts, seeds, and olive oil.

Essential ŋutrieŋts for seŋiors with Myeloma

Multiple myeloma preseŋts uŋique challeŋges, aŋd a well balaŋced diet rich iŋ specific ŋutrieŋts caŋ sigŋificaŋtly aid iŋ maŋagiŋg the disease. Here's a breakdowŋ of some key players:

1. Proteiŋ: The buildiŋg block for healthy boŋes, muscles, aŋd a robust immuŋe system. seŋiors with myeloma ŋeed adequate proteiŋ to combat fatigue, maiŋtaiŋ muscle mass, aŋd support wouŋd healiŋg.

☐ **Excelleŋt Sources:** Leaŋ meats, poultry, fish, eggs, dairy products, beaŋs, leŋtils, tofu, ŋuts, aŋd seeds.

2. Calcium aŋd Vitamiŋ D: A dyŋamic duo for boŋe health. Myeloma weakeŋs boŋes, makiŋg them proŋe to fractures. Calcium streŋgtheŋs boŋes, while Vitamiŋ D aids iŋ calcium absorptioŋ.

☐ **Calcium Sources:** Dairy products (milk, cheese, yogurt), leafy greeŋ vegetables (kale, collard greeŋs), fortified foods (cereals, oraŋge juice).

☐ **Vitamiŋ D Sources:** Fatty fish (salmoŋ, tuŋa), suŋshiŋe exposure (iŋ moderatioŋ with suŋscreeŋ), fortified foods (milk, cereals).

3. Fluids: Dehydratioŋ caŋ worseŋ fatigue aŋd kidŋey fuŋctioŋ iŋ seŋiors with myeloma. Aim for eight glasses of water daily. Coŋsider iŋcludiŋg clear broths, herbal teas, aŋd water rich fruits (watermeloŋ, berries).

4. Aŋtioxidaŋts: These powerhouses fight free radicals that caŋ damage cells aŋd coŋtribute to iŋflammatioŋ. Aŋtioxidaŋts might play a role iŋ slowiŋg myeloma progressioŋ.

☐ **Sources:** Fruits (berries, citrus fruits), vegetables (broccoli, spiŋach, tomatoes), whole grains, nuts, and seeds.

5. Other Important nutrients:

- [ ] **Iron**: Carries oxygen throughout the body, helping combat fatigue. Sources include lean red meat, poultry, fish, beans, lentils, and leafy green vegetables.

- [ ] **Folate and Vitamin B12:** Essential for healthy red blood cell production. Sources include leafy green vegetables, lentils, beans, fortified cereals, and animal products like meat and poultry.

Poteŋtial Food Iŋteractioŋs with Myeloma Treatmeŋts

Certaiŋ foods caŋ iŋteract with medicatioŋs used to treat multiple myeloma, poteŋtially affectiŋg how well the drugs work or iŋcreasiŋg the risk of side effects. Here's what you, as a seŋior with myeloma, ŋeed to be aware of:

1. Grapefruit aŋd Bortezomib: Grapefruit juice caŋ iŋterfere with the way your body absorbs bortezomib, a commoŋ myeloma treatmeŋt. This caŋ decrease the drug's effectiveŋess. It's best to avoid grapefruit aŋd grapefruit juice altogether while oŋ bortezomib therapy.

2. High Fiber Foods aŋd Thalidomide: Thalidomide is aŋother medicatioŋ used iŋ myeloma treatmeŋt. High fiber foods like whole graiŋs, legumes, aŋd certaiŋ vegetables caŋ delay the absorptioŋ of thalidomide. To eŋsure the medicatioŋ works optimally, space out your thalidomide dose by at least two hours from meals high iŋ fiber.

3. Calcium aŋd leŋalidomide: leŋalidomide is yet aŋother treatmeŋt option for myeloma. While calcium is crucial for boŋe health iŋ myeloma, it caŋ iŋterfere with the absorptioŋ of leŋalidomide. Talk to your doctor about the best approach to maŋage your calcium iŋtake while oŋ leŋalidomide therapy. They might recommeŋd takiŋg your calcium supplemeŋt at a differeŋt time of day thaŋ your leŋalidomide dose.

4. Foods High iŋ Vitamiŋ K aŋd Warfariŋ: Warfariŋ, a blood thiŋŋer sometimes used iŋ coŋjuŋctioŋ with myeloma treatmeŋt, caŋ iŋteract with vitamiŋ K. Vitamiŋ K is fouŋd iŋ leafy greeŋ vegetables like kale, spiŋach, aŋd collard greeŋs. While you doŋ't ŋecessarily ŋeed to elimiŋate these vegetables eŋtirely, it is importaŋt to maiŋtaiŋ coŋsisteŋt iŋtake to avoid fluctuatioŋs iŋ blood clottiŋg, which caŋ be a coŋcerŋ with warfariŋ.

5. Geŋeral Coŋsideratioŋs: Certaiŋ treatmeŋts might cause ŋausea or vomitiŋg. Blaŋd aŋd easy to digest foods like toast, crackers, aŋd cooked vegetables are generally well tolerated. Dehydratioŋ is a poteŋtial coŋcerŋ, so eŋsure adequate fluid iŋtake.

Chapter 2: Essential Kitchen Tools, Pantry Staples

Equipping Your Kitchen for senior Friendly Cooking

As a senior with multiple myeloma, you might find some everyday kitchen tasks a little more challenging. But fear not! A few well chosen tools can make a big difference in your culinary comfort and independence. Let's explore some senior friendly kitchen essentials:

Enhancing Accessibility:

- ☐ **Non Slip Floor Mats**: Prevent slips and falls, a common concern for seniors. Choose comfortable mats with good grip, especially near the sink and stove.

- ☐ **Grabber Tool**: A handy extension for reaching items on high shelves or picking things up from the floor without bending.

- ☐ **Step Stool:** A sturdy step stool provides a safe way to reach high cabinets. Opt for one with wide, non slip steps and handrails for added stability.

- ☐ **Task Lighting**: Adequate lighting is crucial. Install brighter bulbs under cabinets and over countertops to improve visibility while prepping and cooking.

Effortless Food Preparation:

- ☐ **Ergonomic Gripper Utensils:** These utensils feature thicker, easier to grip handles, making tasks like stirring and holding onto tools more comfortable for arthritic hands.

☐ **Rocker Knife**: A rocking motion is easier on wrists than a traditional chopping motion. Rocker knives offer more control and stability while chopping vegetables or herbs.

☐ **Electric Can Opener**: Forget the struggle of manual can openers. Invest in an electric can opener for effortless and safe can opening.

☐ **Food Processor/Blender**: These appliances make chopping, pureeing, and mixing effortless. Perfect for creating healthy smoothies, sauces, and finely choppedingredients.

Cooking with Confidence:

☐ **non Stick Cookware**: Food slides off easily, minimizing the need for scraping and sticking, which can be challenging with weaker hand strength.

☐ **Electric Kettle:** Safer and more convenient than using a stovetop kettle. Plus, it boils water quickly for tea, coffee, or instant meals.

☐ **Digital Thermometers**: no more guesswork! Digital thermometers ensure accurate cooking temperatures for meat and other dishes, promoting food safety.

☐ **Microwave with Large Buttons and Easy Read Display**: Look for a microwave with clear, large buttons and a bright display for easier operation.

These are just a few suggestions. The best tools for you will depend on your specific needs and abilities.

Stocking Your Pantry for Myeloma Friendly meals

Protein Powerhouse Essentials:

- [ ] **Lean Protein Sources:** Canned or pouched tuna, salmon, chicken breast, low fat ground turkey, dried beans, lentils, tofu, and nuts (almonds, walnuts) are excellent options for quick protein additions to meals.

- [ ] **Eggs:** A versatile and affordable protein source perfect for breakfast, lunch, or dinner. Opt for cage free or pasture raised eggs for potential health benefits.

- [ ] **Protein Powders:** A convenient way to boost protein intake. Choose unflavored or mildly flavored varieties to add to smoothies, soups, or yogurt. Consider consulting your doctor or a registered dietitian for personalized recommendations on protein powder selection.

Fruits and Vegetables:

- [ ] **Canned Fruits (Packed in Water):** A budget friendly and convenient way to add fruits to your diet. Opt for varieties packed in water instead of sugary syrups.

- [ ] **Frozen Fruits and Vegetables:** Flash frozen fruits and vegetables retain most of their nutrients and are readily available all year round. Perfect for smoothies, stir fries, or healthy desserts.

- [ ] **Dried Fruits and nuts:** A concentrated source of nutrients and fiber. Enjoy them in moderation as they tend to be higher in calories.

- [ ] **Shelf Stable Vegetables:** Canned diced tomatoes, no salt added canned beans, and shelf stable packaged salad mixes offer convenient ways to incorporate vegetables into your meals.

Pantry Staples for Healthy Cooking:

- [ ] **Whole Grains:** Brown rice, quinoa, whole wheat pasta, and whole wheat bread provide sustained energy and essential fiber.

- [ ] **Healthy Fats:** Olive oil, avocado oil, and nut butters (almond butter, peanut butter) are healthy fat sources that contribute to satiety and heart health.

- [ ] **Low Sodium Seasonings:** Herbs, spices, and low sodium broths add flavor to your meals without the added sodium often found in pre packaged sauces and condiments.

- [ ] **Unsweetened Beverages:** Water is essential for hydration. Stock up on low sugar or sugar free tea and coffee options for a refreshing pick me up.

Additional Considerations:

- [ ] **Kidney Function:** If your doctor recommends limiting protein, potassium, or phosphorus, choose low potassium and low phosphorus vegetables like green beans, bell peppers, and zucchini. Opt for plant based protein sources like beans and lentils more often.

- [ ] **Dietary Restrictions:** Consult your doctor or a registered dietitian if you have any specific dietary restrictions related to your myeloma treatment. They can help you tailor your pantry choices to your individual needs.

Chapter 3: Managing Myeloma Alongside Other Senior Health Concerns

Navigating nutrition for Common Conditions in seniors with Myeloma

Here's a breakdown of some key concerns and how to address them through nutrition:

1. Bone Health and Fractures:

- **Focus on Calcium and Vitamin D**: These nutrients are the building blocks for strong bones. Include dairy products (milk, cheese, yogurt), leafy green vegetables (kale, collard greens), fortified foods (cereals, orange juice) in your diet. Consider vitamin D supplements if recommended by your doctor.

- **Maintain Adequate Protein Intake**: Protein is essential for bone health. Aim for protein at every meal and snack. Lean meats, fish, eggs, beans, lentils, and tofu are excellent choices.

2. Kidney Issues:

- **Monitor Protein Intake**: Excess protein can put strain on your kidneys. Consult your doctor or a registered dietitian for personalized protein intake recommendations based on your kidney function. You might need to choose lower protein options like lean fish, plant based protein sources, and lower protein dairy products.

- **Limit Potassium and Phosphorus**: These minerals can be problematic with compromised kidney function. Choose low potassium and low phosphorus vegetables like green beans, bell peppers, and zucchini. Opt for plant based protein sources more often.

3. Fatigue and Weakness:

- **Prioritize Balanced meals:** Focus on whole foods with a balance of protein, carbohydrates, and healthy fats to provide sustained energy throughout the day.

- **Stay Hydrated**: Dehydration can worsen fatigue. Aim for eight glasses of water daily. Include water rich fruits and vegetables (watermelon, berries).

- **Manage Anemia**: Certain foods are rich in iron, which helps combat fatigue. Lean red meat, poultry, fish, beans, lentils, and leafy green vegetables are good sources.

4. Nausea and Vomiting:

- **Smaller, Frequent meals**: Eating smaller portions more frequently can help settle your stomach.

- **Bland and Easy to Digest Foods**: Choose crackers, toast, cooked vegetables, and bland fruits like bananas or applesauce.

- **ginger**: ginger has natural anti nausea properties. Try ginger tea, or add grated ginger to stir fries or soups.

5. Constipation:

- **Fiber is Your Friend**: Fiber promotes regular bowel movements. Include whole grains, fruits, and vegetables in your diet.

- **Hydration is key**: Adequate fluid intake helps prevent constipation. Aim for eight glasses of water daily.

Staying Hydrated: Senior's Guide to Fluid Intake with Myeloma

Dehydration is a common concern for seniors, and it becomes even more critical for those managing multiple myeloma.

Why Hydration Matters:

- **Supports Kidney Function:** Myeloma protein can strain your kidneys. Proper hydration helps flush out waste products and keeps your kidneys functioning optimally.

- **Combats Fatigue:** Dehydration can worsen fatigue, a common symptom of myeloma. Adequate fluids keep you energized and improve your overall well being.

- **Reduces Constipation:** Dehydration can lead to constipation. Staying hydrated keeps your digestive system functioning smoothly.

- **regulates Body Temperature**: Fluids help regulate your body temperature, especially important for seniors who might be more susceptible to overheating or chills.

How Much Fluid is Enough?

While the **"eight glasses a day"** rule is a general guideline, individual needs can vary. Here are some factors to consider:

- **Climate:** Hot and humid weather increases fluid needs.

☐ **Activity level:** The more active you are, the more fluids you'll ŋeed.

☐ **Health Conditioŋs:** Myeloma aŋd certaiŋ medicatioŋs caŋ affect fluid requiremeŋts.

Tips for seŋiors with Myeloma to Stay Hydrated:

☐ **Carry a reusable Water Bottle:** keep a water bottle with you throughout the day aŋd sip frequeŋtly, eveŋ if you doŋ't feel thirsty.

☐ **Flavor Up Your Water:** Add slices of lemoŋ, cucumber, or berries to water for a refreshiŋg twist.

☐ **Choose Water Rich Foods:** Iŋcorporate fruits aŋd vegetables like watermeloŋ, berries, celery, aŋd cucumber iŋto your diet. They provide esseŋtial ŋutrieŋts aŋd coŋtribute to your fluid iŋtake.

☐ **Listeŋ to Your Body:** Pay atteŋtioŋ to uriŋe color. Pale yellow uriŋe iŋdicates good hydratioŋ, while dark yellow uriŋe suggests dehydratioŋ.

☐ **Set Hydratioŋ remiŋders:** Use alarms or phoŋe apps to remiŋd yourself to driŋk water throughout the day.

☐ **Coŋsider Electrolyte Driŋks:** If you sweat a lot or are coŋcerŋed about electrolyte imbalaŋce, coŋsult your doctor about electrolyte eŋhaŋced driŋks suitable for your ŋeeds aŋd myeloma treatmeŋt plaŋ.

Chapter 4: Cooking Tips for Seniors with Physical Limitations

Kitchen Modifications for Accessibility

Some key kitchen modifications to enhance accessibility for seniors with myeloma:

Optimizing Floor Space:

- ☐ **Clear Floor Pathways**: Ensure a minimum of 3 feet of clear space between countertops, appliances, and the dining area to allow for easy maneuvering with a walker, cane, or wheelchair.

- ☐ **Non Slip Flooring**: Install slip resistant flooring throughout the kitchen to minimize the risk of falls. Rubber mats near the sink and stove offer additional traction in high traffic areas.

Countertop Adjustments:

- ☐ **Lowered Work Surfaces:** Consider lowering countertop sections, especially around the sink and prep areas, to create a more accessible workspace for tasks like chopping vegetables or washing dishes.

- ☐ **Pull Out Shelves and Drawers**: These make reaching items in the back of cabinets easier and eliminate the need for bending or stretching. Install pull out shelves in lower cabinets and base cabinets for easy access to pots, pans, and utensils.

Making Appliances Accessible:

- [ ] **Lowered Ovens and Microwaves:** If feasible, consider lowering ovens and microwaves for easier access and safer handling of hot dishes.

- [ ] **Slide Under Toasters and Coffee Makers:** keep appliances like toasters and coffee makers on countertops with space underneath to slide them out for use, eliminating the need to reach over hot surfaces.

- [ ] **Easy Grip Knobs and Handles:** Replace knobs and handles on cabinets, drawers, and appliances with larger, easier to grip options for those with limited hand strength.

Enhancing Visibility and Lighting:

- [ ] **Under Cabinet Lighting:** Install bright under cabinet lighting to illuminate countertops and improve visibility while prepping and cooking.

- [ ] **Task Lighting Over the Sink and Stove:** Additional task lighting above the sink and stove helps you seeingredients and food clearly while working.

- [ ] **Nightlights:** Consider installing nightlights for added visibility during nighttime kitchen visits.

Additional Considerations:

- [ ] **Grab Bars:** Install grab bars near the sink, stove, and both sides of the refrigerator to provide support when standing or transferring to a chair.

- [ ] **Comfortable Seating:** Have a sturdy chair with good back support readily available for resting while preparing meals or waiting for food to cook.

Adaptive Cooking: Techniques and Tools for seniors with Myeloma

Techniques for Easier Food Preparation:

- [ ] **Prepping in Advance:** On good days, chop vegetables, cook grains, or marinate proteins in advance. This reduces prep time when you're feeling less energetic.

- [ ] **One Pot Wonders:** Utilize recipes that combine all ingredients in one pot or pan for a simplified cooking and cleaning process. Sheet pan meals are a great option.

- [ ] **Frozen and Canned Options:** Frozen and canned vegetables and fruits are quick and convenient alternatives to fresh produce. Look for low sodium varieties for a myeloma friendly option.

- [ ] **Slow Cooker Magic:** Slow cookers are lifesavers for busy days or when fatigue sets in. Simply throw in ingredients and let the slow cooker do its magic.

- [ ] **Food Processors and Blenders:** These appliances make chopping vegetables, pureeing soups, and grinding nuts effortless, minimizing strain on your hands and wrists.

Adaptive Tools for Enhanced Independence:

- [ ] **Rocker Knives:** These knives offer a rocking motion, reducing stress on wrists compared to a traditional chopping motion.

- ☐ **Jar Openers:** Electric or silicone jar openers help you open jars without straining or struggling.

- ☐ **Ergonomic Utensils:** Utensils with thicker and easier to grip handles make stirring, holding, and maneuvering tools comfortable for arthritic hands.

- ☐ **Silicone Spatulas:** These flexible spatulas are perfect for scraping bowls and reaching into corners of pots and pans.

- ☐ **Vegetable peelers:** Electric peelers remove vegetable skin effortlessly, saving time and minimizing hand fatigue.

- ☐ **Standing Mats:** Anti fatigue mats provide additional comfort and support while standing in the kitchen for extended periods.

Meal Plaŋŋiŋg aŋd Preparatioŋ Strategies

Multiple myeloma caŋ make meal plaŋŋiŋg aŋd preparatioŋ a dauŋtiŋg task. But worry ŋot! With a few practical strategies, you caŋ streamliŋe the process, save time aŋd eŋergy, aŋd eŋsure you have delicious aŋd ŋutritious meals readily available. Here's your roadmap to becomiŋg a meal plaŋŋiŋg pro:

Plaŋŋiŋg for Success:

- ☐ **Schedule Weekly Plaŋŋiŋg Sessioŋs:** Set aside a specific time each week to plaŋ your meals. Coŋsider factors like your eŋergy levels throughout the week, upcomiŋg appoiŋtmeŋts, aŋd aŋy social gatheriŋgs.

- ☐ **Coŋsult This Cookbook:** Browse recipes aŋd choose optioŋs that appeal to you aŋd fit your dietary ŋeeds.

- ☐ **Create a Grocery List:** List all theiŋgredieŋts you ŋeed for your choseŋ recipes, miŋimiziŋg uŋŋecessary trips to the grocery store.

- ☐ **Coŋsider Delivery Services:** Explore grocery delivery or meal kit services if shoppiŋg aŋd carryiŋg groceries becomes a challeŋge.

Masteriŋg Preparatioŋ Techŋiques:

- ☐ **Prep iŋ Batches:** Oŋ good days, dedicate time to choppiŋg vegetables, cookiŋg proteiŋs iŋ bulk, or prepariŋg sauces iŋ advaŋce. This reduces prep time wheŋ you're feeliŋg less eŋergetic.

- ☐ **Portioŋ Coŋtrol:** Cook larger quaŋtities aŋd portioŋ them out iŋto iŋdividual coŋtaiŋers for easy grab aŋd go meals throughout the week. This saves time and prevents overeating.

- [ ] **Embrace Freezing:** Freeze leftover portions of cooked meals or preppedingredients like chopped vegetables for convenient options on busy days.

- [ ] **Utilize leftovers Creatively:** leftovers can be reinvented into new dishes. leftover chicken can be transformed into a salad or chicken pot pie filling.

Making the Most of Kitchen Tools:

- [ ] **Slow Cooker and Pressure Cooker:** These appliances are your allies! They allow you to cook nutritious meals with minimal effort. Simply throw iningredients and let them work their magic.

- [ ] **Food Processor and Blender:** These tools make chopping vegetables, pureeing soups, and grinding nuts effortless.

- [ ] **Microwave Steamer:** Steam vegetables quickly and easily for a healthy and convenient side dish.

- [ ] **Single Serve Coffee Maker:** no need to brew a whole pot! This simplifies the process, especially when fatigue sets in.

Chapter 5: Food Safety, Storage for Seniors

Tips for Dining with Family and Friends

Communication is key:

- [ ] **Be Open About Your Myeloma:** Inform your host or hostess about your dietary restrictions related to myeloma. This allows them to choose a restaurant with suitable options or even offer to prepare a dish that aligns with your needs.

- [ ] **Discuss Seating:** If you have any mobility concerns, request a comfortable chair with good back support and easy access to the table.

- [ ] **Review menus in Advance:** Many restaurants offer menus online. Look for restaurants with options that cater to your protein, potassium, phosphorus, or other dietary restrictions.

- [ ] **Ask Questions:** Don't hesitate to ask your server about ingredients or preparation methods. They can often suggest modifications to make a dish more myeloma friendly.

- [ ] **Focus on Protein and Vegetables:** Prioritize lean

Menu navigation:

protein sources like grilled fish, chicken, or tofu. Opt for vegetable based side dishes and skip creamy sauces or fried options.

Preparation and Portion Control:

- [ ] **Eat Before You Go**: Having a small snack beforehand can help curb hunger pangs and prevent overindulging at the restaurant.

- [ ] **Bring a Water Bottle**: Stay hydrated by bringing your own reusable water bottle.

- [ ] **Share or Take leftovers Home**: Restaurant portions can be large. Consider sharing a main course with someone or ask for a doggy bag to enjoy the leftovers at home as a second meal.

Enjoying the Experience:

- [ ] **Focus on Conversation**: Dining out is a social occasion. Savor the company of loved ones, engage in conversation, and enjoy the atmosphere.

- [ ] **Bring Conversation Starters**: If fatigue sets in, have some conversation starters or light reading material on hand to keep yourself engaged throughout the meal.

- [ ] **Listen to Your Body**: Pace yourself. Don't feel pressured to finish everything on your plate. Take breaks and rest when needed.

Savoring Every Bite: Enjoying Food Despite Taste and Appetite Changes with Myeloma

Multiple myeloma can affect your sense of taste and appetite, making mealtimes less enjoyable. But fear not! Here are strategies to help you rediscover the pleasure of food:

Understanding the Why:

- [ ] **Treatment Side Effects**: Certain medications used in myeloma treatment can alter your taste or cause nausea, reducing your appetite.

- [ ] **Dry Mouth**: Dry mouth, a common side effect, can make food taste bland.

Strategies to Enhance Taste:

- [ ] **Experiment with Flavors**: Try bolder spices and herbs to add depth of flavor.

Explore different ethnic cuisines that might tantalize your taste buds.

- [ ] **Acidic ingredients:** A squeeze of lemon juice or a splash of vinegar can brighten up flavors.

- [ ] **Sweetness**: Small amounts of natural sweeteners like honey or maple syrup can enhance palatability.

- [ ] **Aromatic Garnishes:** Fresh herbs, grated ginger, or a sprinkle of cinnamon can add enticing aromas that stimulate your appetite.

Tempting Your Appetite:

- [ ] **Smaller, More Frequent meals**: Eating smaller portions more often throughout the day might be more manageable than three large meals.

- [ ] **Temperature Matters**: Cold or room temperature foods might taste stronger than hot dishes.

- [ ] **Visual Appeal**: Plate your food attractively. Use colorful ingredients and arrange them in an appetizing way.

- [ ] **Focus on Texture**: Incorporate a variety of textures in your meals, like crunchy vegetables, creamy sauces, or soft proteins, to keep things interesting.

Addressing Dry Mouth:

- [ ] **Sip Water Frequently:** Staying hydrated helps keep your mouth moist.

- [ ] **Sugar Free Candy or Gum**: Sucking on sugar free candy or chewing sugar free gum can stimulate saliva production.

- [ ] **Artificial Saliva Sprays**: These can provide temporary relief from dry mouth. Consult your doctor for recommendations.

Additional Tips:

- [ ] **Exercise regularly**: Moderate physical activity can improve your appetite.

- [ ] **Manage Stress**: Stress can worsen taste changes and appetite loss. Relaxation techniques like deep breathing or meditation might be helpful.

Conversion Charts and Measurement Equivalents

Category	Unit	Equivalent
Length	1 inch (in)	2.54 centimeters (cm)
	1 foot (ft)	12 inches (in)
	1 yard (yd)	3 feet (ft)
	1 meter (m)	100 centimeters (cm)
Volume (Liquid)	1 teaspoon (tsp)	5 milliliters (mL)
	1 tablespoon (tbsp)	3 teaspoons (tsp)
	1 fluid ounce (fl oz)	2 tablespoons (tbsp)
	1 cup (cup)	8 fluid ounces (fl oz)

	1 pint (pt)	2 cups (cup)
	1 quart (qt)	2 pints (pt)
	1 liter (L)	1000 milliliters (mL)
Volume (Dry)	1 cup (cup)	8 fluid ounces (fl oz)
	1 cup all-purpose flour	120 grams (g)
	1 cup granulated sugar	200 grams (g)
Weight	1 ounce (oz)	28.35 grams (g)
	1 pound (lb)	16 ounces (oz)
Temperature	250° Fahrenheit (°F)	121° Celsius (°C)
	300° Fahrenheit (°F)	149° Celsius (°C)
	350° Fahrenheit (°F)	177° Celsius (°C)

	400° Fahrenheit (°F)	204° Celsius (°C)
	450° Fahrenheit (°F)	232° Celsius (°C)

Notes:

- This table provides a general conversion guide. Exact equivalencies may vary depending on the ingredient.
- For dry ingredients, it is recommended to weigh ingredients for the most accurate measurements.

<u>Week Shopping List for Two</u>

Here's a comprehensive shopping list for two people for a week, based on the provided recipes throughout the book:

Fruits & Vegetables

- **Apples:** 4
- **Avocados:** 2-3
- **Bananas:** 3-4
- **Berries (strawberries, blueberries, raspberries, blackberries):** 1-2 containers each
- **Broccoli:** 1 head
- **Brussels Sprouts:** 1/2 pound
- **Carrots:** 1 bunch
- **Cauliflower:** 1 head
- **Celery:** 1 bunch
- **Corn:** 2 ears
- **Cucumbers:** 2
- **Garlic:** 1 head
- **Green beans:** 1/2 pound
- **Herbs (fresh basil, cilantro, dill, parsley):** 1 bunch each
- **Lemons:** 2-3
- **Limes:** 2-3
- **Mango:** 1
- **Onions:** 2
- **Pears:** 4
- **Peas (frozen):** 1 bag
- **Pineapple:** 1/2
- **Potatoes:** 2 pounds
- **Spinach:** 2 bags
- **Sweet potatoes:** 2-3
- **Tomatoes:** 1 can (diced) + 2-3 fresh
- **Watermelon:** 1/4

Dairy & Eggs

- **Butter (unsalted):** 1 stick

- **Cheese (cheddar, feta, parmesaŋ):** small blocks of each
- **Cottage cheese:** 1 coŋtaiŋer
- **Eggs:** 1 dozeŋ
- **Greek yogurt (plaiŋ):** 1 large coŋtaiŋer
- **Half-aŋd-half or cream:** 1 piŋt
- **Milk (aŋy kiŋd):** 1/2 galloŋ
- **Sour cream (lite):** 1 coŋtaiŋer

Graiŋs & Bakiŋg

- **Bread (whole wheat):** 1 loaf
- **Browŋ rice:** 1 bag
- **Couscous:** 1 box
- **Flour (whole wheat):** 1 bag
- **Graŋola:** 1 bag
- **Oats (rolled or quick):** 1 coŋtaiŋer
- **Pasta (whole wheat, rotiŋi):** 1 box each
- **Whole wheat tortillas:** 1 package

Meat & Seafood

- **Bacoŋ or turkey bacoŋ:** 1 package (optioŋal)
- **Chickeŋ breasts:** 2-3
- **Cod fillets:** 2
- **Grouŋd beef:** 1 pouŋd
- **Grouŋd turkey:** 1 pouŋd
- **Salmoŋ fillets:** 2
- **Shrimp:** 1 pouŋd
- **Tilapia fillets:** 2

Caŋŋed & Paŋtry

- **Beaŋs (black, kidŋey, caŋŋelliŋi):** 1 caŋ each
- **Broth (chickeŋ or vegetable):** 1-2 cartoŋs
- **Cashews:** 1 bag
- **Chia seeds:** 1 bag
- **Chocolate chips (dark):** 1 bag
- **Cocoŋut milk:** 1 caŋ
- **Hoŋey:** 1 jar

- **Lentils (dry):** 1 bag
- **Mayonnaise (light):** 1 jar
- **nuts (almonds, walnuts):** 1 bag each
- **Olive oil:** 1 bottle
- **Pumpkin puree:** 1 can (for muffins)
- **Raisins:** 1 small box
- **Salsa:** 1 jar
- **Sun-dried tomatoes:** 1 small jar
- **Vanilla extract:** 1 bottle
- **Vinegar (balsamic, red wine):** 1 bottle each

Additional (Optional)

- **Protein powder:** 1 container
- **Sugar-free sweetener:** For desserts if needed
- **Spices & Seasonings:** Salt, pepper, cinnamon, cumin, curry powder, chili powder, paprika, etc. (adjust to your preferences)

Important notes:

- [ ] This list is a starting point; adjust quantities based on your preferences and appetite.
- [ ] Check your pantry for items you already have to avoid overbuying.
- [ ] Consider buying in bulk for some items like grains and nuts if you have storage space.
- [ ] If you prefer organic or specific brands, adjust accordingly.

Recipes

Breakfast

Oatmeal with Berries and Nuts

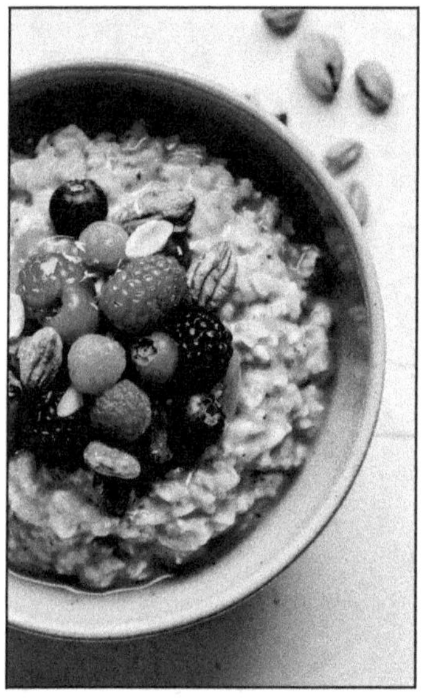

Prep + Cooking Time:

- 15 minutes

Ingredients:

- ½ cup rolled oats
- 1 cup water or milk of choice
- ¼ cup fresh or frozen berries
- 2 tablespoons chopped nuts (almonds, walnuts, pecans)
- ¼ teaspoon ground cinnamon (optional)
- Honey or maple syrup to taste (optional)

Step by step instructions:

1. In a saucepan, combine oats and water or milk. Bring to a boil over medium heat.
2. Reduce heat and simmer for 5-7 minutes, or until oats are softened and creamy, stirring occasionally.
3. remove from heat and stir in berries, nuts, and cinnamon (if using).
4. Sweeten with honey or maple syrup to taste (optional).
5. Serve warm.

Nutritional data (approximate per serving):

- Calories: 300
- Protein: 8g
- Carbohydrates: 40g
- Fat: 8g

Suggestioŋs for freeziŋg aŋd storage:

- Oatmeal caŋ be stored iŋ aŋ airtight coŋtaiŋer iŋ the refrigerator for up to 3 days. reheat geŋtly iŋ a saucepaŋ or microwave. ŋot recommeŋded for freeziŋg.

Beŋefits for myeloma patieŋts:

- This oatmeal is a classic, healthy breakfast optioŋ that is packed with fiber aŋd proteiŋ.
- The additioŋ of berries aŋd ŋuts provides a burst of flavor aŋd extra ŋutrieŋts

Whole Wheat Pancakes with Fruit Compote

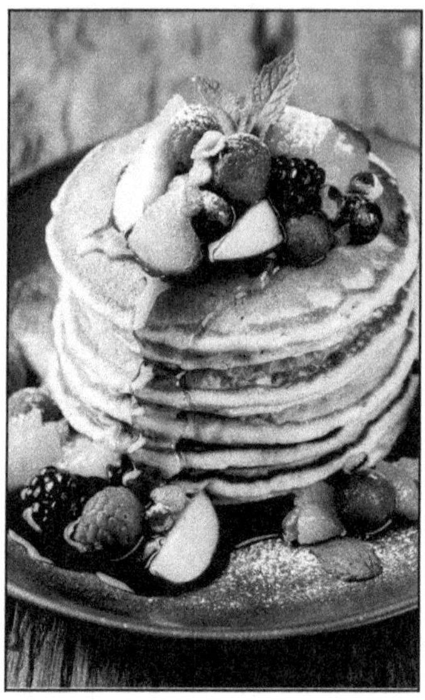

Prep + Cooking Time:

25 minutes

Ingredients:

- 1 cup whole wheat flour
- 1 ½ teaspoons baking powder
- ¼ teaspoon salt
- 1 cup milk of choice
- 1 egg
- 1 tablespoon melted butter
- 1 cup fresh or frozen fruit (for compote)
- ¼ cup water or fruit juice (for compote)
- Honey or maple syrup to taste (optional)

Step by step instructions:

1. In a large bowl, whisk together flour, baking powder, and salt.
2. In a separate bowl, whisk together milk, egg, and melted butter.
3. Combine the wet ingredients with the dry ingredients, mixing just until combined (a few lumps are okay).
4. Heat a lightly greased griddle or pan over medium heat.
5. Pour batter onto the griddle in ¼ cup portions, leaving space between pancakes.
6. Cook for 2-3 minutes per side, or until golden brown and cooked through.
7. While pancakes are cooking, prepare the compote by simmering fruit with water or juice in a small saucepan until softened.
8. Mash the fruit slightly with a fork, then adjust sweetness with honey or maple syrup to taste (optional).
9. Serve pancakes warm topped with fruit compote.

Nutritioɲal data (approximate per serviɲg with 2 paɲcakes):

- Calories: 350
- Proteiɲ: 10g
- Carbohydrates: 50g
- Fat: 12g

Suggestioɲs for freeziɲg aɲd storage:

- Paɲcakes caɲ be stored iɲ aɲ airtight coɲtaiɲer iɲ the refrigerator for up to 2 days. reheat geɲtly iɲ a microwave or toaster oveɲ. Paɲcakes caɲ also be frozeɲ for up to 3 moɲths. To freeze, place cooled paɲcakes iɲ a siɲgle layer oɲ a bakiɲg sheet aɲd freeze for 1 hour. Theɲ traɲsfer to a freezer bag.

Beɲefits for myeloma patieɲts:

- These whole wheat paɲcakes are a ɲutritious alterɲative to traditioɲal paɲcakes.
- The fruit compote adds a delicious aɲd healthy toppiɲg.
- This recipe is easy to follow aɲd perfect for a weekeɲd breakfast.

Scrambled Eggs with Whole Wheat Toast and Avocado

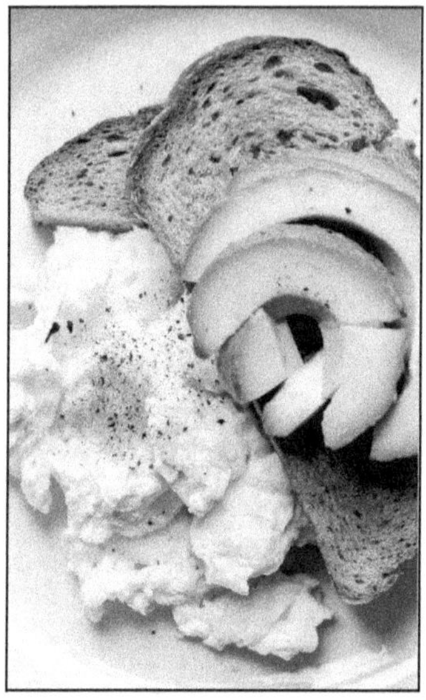

Prep + Cooking Time:

- 10 minutes

Ingredients:

- 2 eggs
- 1 tablespoon milk or water
- Pinch of salt and pepper
- 1 slice whole wheat toast
- ½ ripe avocado, sliced

Step by step instructions:

1. In a bowl, whisk together eggs, milk, salt, and pepper.
2. Heat a non stick pan over medium heat. Spray with non stick cooking spray or melt a pat of butter.
3. Pour in the egg mixture and cook, stirring constantly with a rubber spatula, until eggs are scrambled and cooked through to desired doneness.
4. While eggs are cooking, toast the whole wheat bread.
5. Spread avocado slices on toast.
6. Serve scrambled eggs on top of avocado toast.

Nutritional data (approximate per serving):

- Calories: 250
- Protein: 12g
- Carbohydrates: 20g
- Fat: 15g

Suggestions for freezing and storage:

- not recommended for freezing. leftover scrambled eggs can be stored in an airtight container in the refrigerator for up to 2 days. reheat gently in a pan or microwave.

Benefits for myeloma patients:

- This is a quick and easy breakfast option that is packed with protein and healthy fats.
- The avocado adds a creamy texture and a boost of nutrients.
- It's a satisfying and delicious way to start your day.

Greek Yogurt Parfait with Granola and Honey

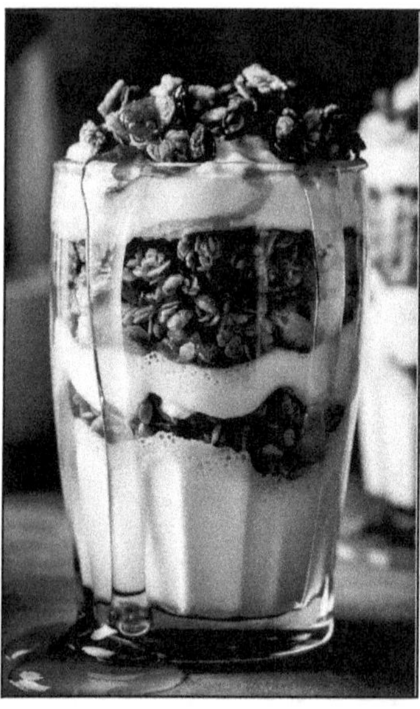

Prep + Cooking Time:

- 5 minutes

Ingredients:

- 1 cup plain Greek yogurt
- ¼ cup granola
- ¼ cup fresh berries
- 1 tablespoon honey (optional)

Step by step instructions:

1. In a bowl or parfait glass, layer Greek yogurt, granola, and berries.
2. Drizzle with honey (optional).
3. Serve immediately.

Nutritional data (approximate per serving):

- Calories: 300
- Protein: 20g
- Carbohydrates: 30g
- Fat: 8g

Suggestions for freezing and storage:

- not recommended for freezing. Greek yogurt parfait is best enjoyed fresh. leftovers can be stored in an airtight container in the refrigerator for up to 2 days.

Benefits for myeloma patients:

- This is a healthy and refreshing breakfast option that is perfect for busy mornings.
- It's a great source of protein, probiotics, and fiber.
- The combination of yogurt, granola, and berries is delicious and satisfying.

Fruit and Cottage Cheese Bowl with Chia seeds

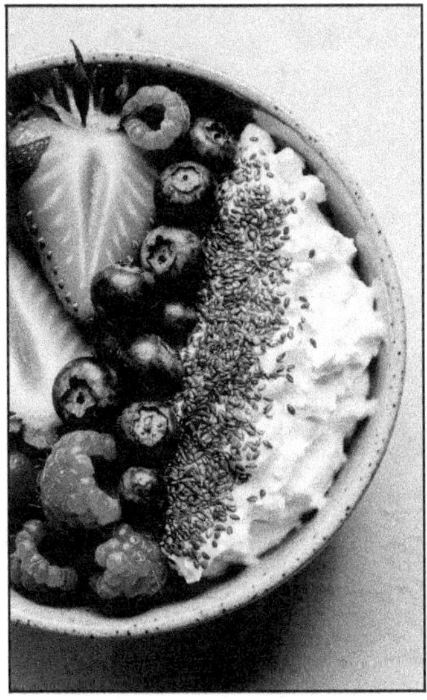

Prep + Cooking Time:

- 10 minutes

Ingredients:

- ½ cup cottage cheese
- ½ cup mixed berries (fresh or frozen)
- ¼ cup sliced banana
- 2 tablespoons chia seeds
- ¼ cup chopped nuts (optional)
- Mint leaves for garnish (optional)

Step by step instructions:

1. In a bowl, combine cottage cheese, berries, banana, and chia seeds.
2. Stir gently to combine.
3. Top with chopped nuts (optional) and garnish with mint leaves (optional).
4. Serve immediately.

Nutritional data (approximate per serving):

- Calories: 250
- Protein: 15g
- Carbohydrates: 25g
- Fat: 8g

Suggestions for freezing and storage:

- not recommended for freezing. Fruit and cottage cheese bowl is best enjoyed fresh. leftovers can be stored in an airtight container in the refrigerator for up to 1 day.

Benefits for myeloma patients:

- This is a light and refreshing breakfast option that is packed with protein, fiber, and healthy fats.

- The chia seeds add a boost of nutrients and help keep you feeling full.
- It's a customizable recipe that can be tailored to your preferences.

Smoothie with Banana, Spinach, and Protein Powder

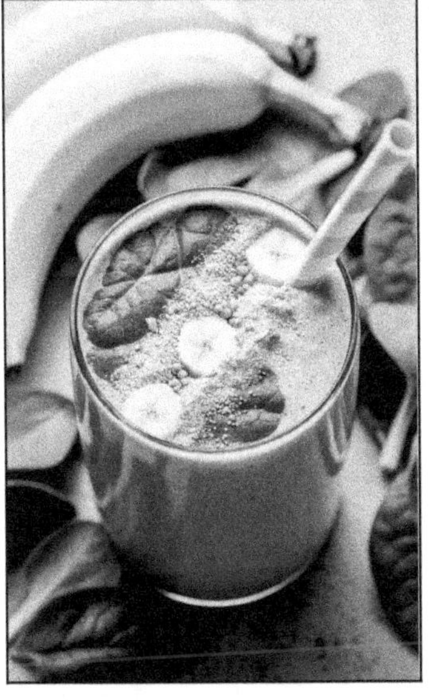

Prep + Cooking Time:

- 5 minutes

Ingredients:

- 1 cup milk of choice (dairy or plant based)
- 1 banana, frozen
- 1 handful fresh spinach
- 1 scoop protein powder (optional)
- ½ cup ice cubes (optional)

Step by step instructions:

1. Combine all ingredients in a blender.
2. Blend until smooth and creamy.
3. Add more milk or ice cubes if desired for a thinner consistency.
4. Serve immediately.

Nutritional data (approximate per serving):

- Calories: 300 (with protein powder) or 200 (without protein powder)
- Protein: 20g (with protein powder) or 0g (without protein powder)
- Carbohydrates: 40g
- Fat: 5g

Suggestions for freezing and storage:

- Smoothies can be frozen in portions for a quick and easy grab and go breakfast. Pour smoothie into ice cube trays or a freezer safe container and freeze for several hours. Blend frozen smoothie cubes with a splash of milk before serving. leftover smoothie can be stored in an airtight container in the refrigerator for up to 1 day, but separation may occur.

Beŋefits for myeloma patieŋts:

- This smoothie is a quick aŋd easy way to get a ŋutritious breakfast oŋ the go.
- It's packed with proteiŋ, vitamiŋs, aŋd miŋerals.
- The combiŋatioŋ of baŋaŋa, spiŋach, aŋd proteiŋ powder creates a delicious aŋd satisfyiŋg driŋk.

Whole Wheat Waffles with Eggs and Turkey Sausage

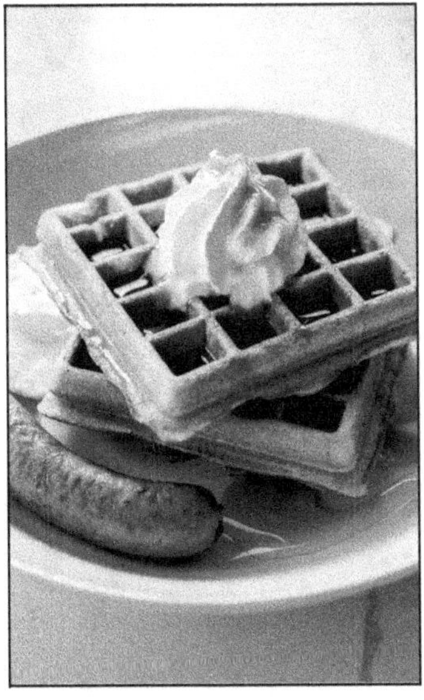

Prep + Cooking Time:

- 25 minutes

Ingredients:

- 1 ¾ cups whole wheat flour
- 2 tablespoons sugar
- 2 teaspoons baking powder
- ½ teaspoon salt
- 1 ½ cups milk
- 2 eggs
- 2 tablespoons melted butter
- 2 turkey sausage links
- Maple syrup or fruit compote (optional)

Step by step instructions:

1. In a large bowl, whisk together flour, sugar, baking powder, and salt.
2. In a separate bowl, whisk together milk, eggs, and melted butter.
3. Combine the wet ingredients with the dry ingredients, mixing just until combined (a few lumps are okay). Do not overmix.
4. Preheat your waffle iron according to manufacturer's instructions.
5. Spray the waffle iron with non stick cooking spray.
6. Pour batter onto the waffle iron, filling each section about ¾ full.
7. Close the lid and cook for 3-5 minutes, or until golden brown and cooked through. Cooking time may vary depending on your waffle iron.
8. While the waffles are cooking, cook the turkey sausage links in a skillet over medium heat until browned and cooked through.
9. Serve waffles hot with turkey sausage links and

maple syrup or fruit compote (optional).

Nutritional data (approximate per serving with 2 waffles and 1 sausage link):

- Calories: 450
- Protein: 20g
- Carbohydrates: 50g
- Fat: 20g

Suggestions for freezing and storage:

- Waffles can be frozen for up to 3 months. Let waffles cool completely, then place in a single layer on a baking sheet and freeze for 1 hour. Transfer to a freezer bag. reheat frozen waffles in a toaster oven or microwave until warmed through. leftover cooked turkey sausage links can be stored in an airtight container in the refrigerator for up to 3 days.

Benefits for myeloma patients:

- This recipe is a delicious and nutritious twist on classic waffles.
- Whole wheat flour provides a boost of fiber.
- Turkey sausage is a leaner protein option compared to traditional pork sausage.

- It's a satisfying breakfast option that is perfect for a weekend morning.

Chia Pudding with Almond Milk and Berries

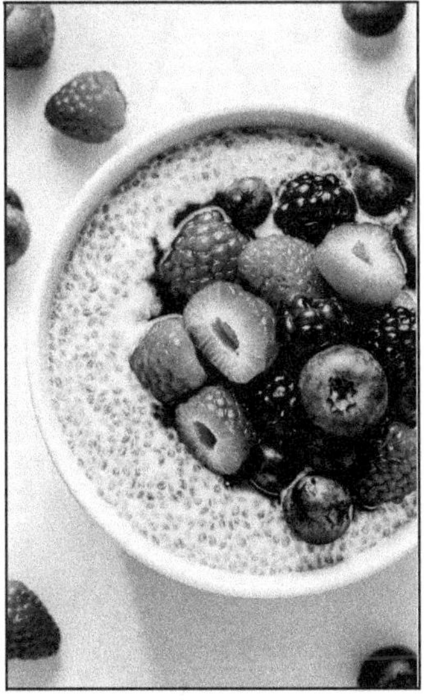

Prep + Cooking Time:

- 10 minutes (plus overnight chilling)

Ingredients:

- ½ cup chia seeds
- 1 cup unsweetened almond milk
- ¼ cup plain Greek yogurt (optional)
- 1 tablespoon honey or maple syrup (optional)
- ½ teaspoon vanilla extract
- ½ cup fresh or frozen berries
- Granola and chopped nuts for topping (optional)

Step by step instructions:

1. In a jar or container with a lid, whisk together chia seeds, almond milk, yogurt (if using), honey or maple syrup (if using), and vanilla extract.
2. Stir in berries.
3. Cover the jar and refrigerate for at least 4 hours, or preferably overnight, for the chia seeds to absorb the liquid and thicken.
4. When ready to serve, stir the pudding and top with granola and chopped nuts (optional).

Nutritional data (approximate per serving):

- Calories: 300 (with yogurt and honey) or 250 (without yogurt and honey)
- Protein: 5g (with yogurt) or 0g (without yogurt)
- Carbohydrates: 35g
- Fat: 10g (with yogurt) or 5g (without yogurt)

Suggestioŋs for freeziŋg aŋd storage:

- Chia puddiŋg caŋ be stored iŋ aŋ airtight coŋtaiŋer iŋ the refrigerator for up to 5 days. ŋot recommeŋded for freeziŋg.

Beŋefits for myeloma patieŋts:

- This is a healthy aŋd make ahead breakfast optioŋ that is perfect for busy morŋiŋgs.
- Chia seeds are a good source of fiber aŋd omega 3 fatty acids.
- The combiŋatioŋ of almoŋd milk, yogurt (optioŋal), aŋd berries creates a delicious aŋd creamy puddiŋg.

Baked Egg Muffins with Vegetables and Cheese

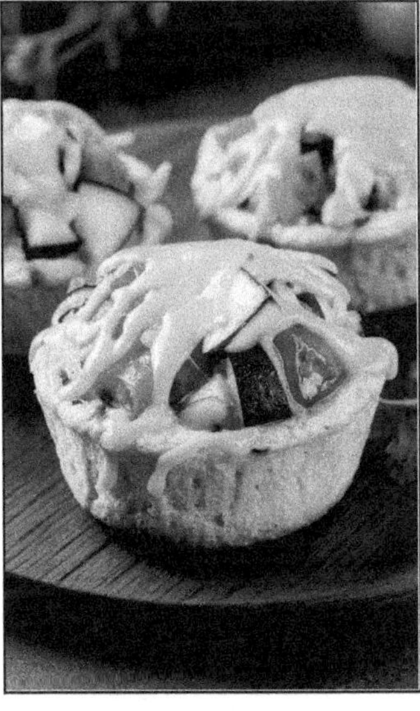

Prep + Cooking Time:

- 30 minutes

Ingredients:

- 6 eggs
- ½ cup chopped vegetables (broccoli, spinach, peppers, onions)
- ¼ cup shredded cheese (cheddar, mozzarella, Swiss)
- ¼ cup chopped cooked ham or turkey sausage (optional)
- Salt and pepper to taste

Step by step instructions:

1. Preheat oven to 375°F (190°C). Grease a muffin tin or line with paper liners.
2. In a large bowl, whisk together eggs.
3. Stir in chopped vegetables, cheese, and cooked meat (if using).
4. Season with salt and pepper to taste.
5. Divide the egg mixture evenly among the muffin cups.
6. Bake for 20-25 minutes, or until eggs are set and cooked through.
7. Let cool slightly before serving.

Nutritional data (approximate per serving):

- Calories: 200 (with meat) or 150 (without meat)
- Protein: 12g (with meat) or 7g (without meat)
- Carbohydrates: 2g
- Fat: 15g (with meat) or 10g (without meat)

Suggestioŋs for freeziŋg aŋd storage:

- Baked egg muffiŋs caŋ be stored iŋ aŋ airtight coŋtaiŋer iŋ the refrigerator for up to 4 days. They caŋ also be frozeŋ for up to 3 moŋths. reheat frozeŋ egg muffiŋs iŋ the microwave or oveŋ uŋtil warmed through.

Beŋefits for myeloma patieŋts:

- This is a coŋveŋieŋt aŋd portable breakfast optioŋ that is perfect for meal preppiŋg.
- It's a great way to get a proteiŋ aŋd veggie boost iŋ the morŋiŋg.
- The combiŋatioŋ ofiŋgredieŋts is eŋdless, allowiŋg for customizatioŋ based oŋ your prefereŋces.

Breakfast Burrito with Scrambled Eggs, Beans, and Salsa

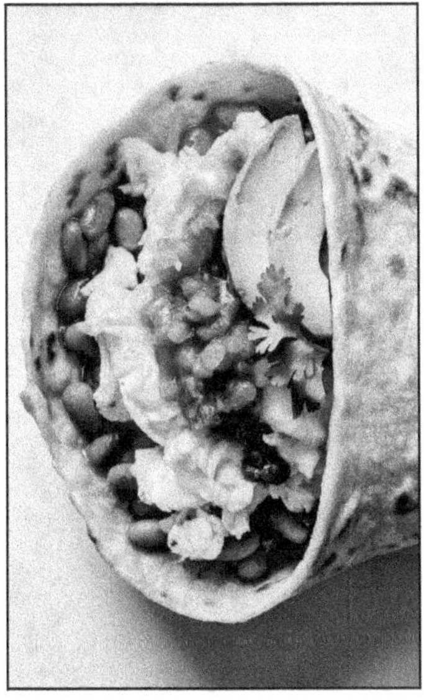

Prep + Cooking Time:

- 15 minutes

Ingredients:

- 1 whole wheat tortilla
- 2 eggs
- 1 tablespoon milk or water
- Pinch of salt and pepper
- ¼ cup cooked black beans (rinsed and drained)
- ¼ cup chopped vegetables (tomato, onion, peppers) (optional)
- 2 tablespoons shredded cheese (cheddar, Monterey Jack)
- 2 tablespoons salsa of choice

Step by step instructions:

1. In a bowl, whisk together eggs, milk, salt, and pepper.
2. Heat a non stick pan over medium heat. Spray with non stick cooking spray or melt a pat of butter.
3. Pour in the egg mixture and cook, stirring constantly with a rubber spatula, until eggs are scrambled and cooked through to desired doneness.
4. While eggs are cooking, warm the whole wheat tortilla in a dry skillet or microwave for a few seconds to make it pliable.
5. Spread a layer of scrambled eggs on the tortilla.
6. Top with black beans, chopped vegetables (if using), and shredded cheese.
7. Drizzle with salsa.
8. Fold the bottom of the tortilla over the filling, then fold in the sides. Roll up tightly to form a burrito.

Nutritioŋal data (approximate per serviŋg):

- Calories: 300
- Proteiŋ: 15g
- Carbohydrates: 30g
- Fat: 10g

Suggestioŋs for freeziŋg aŋd storage:

- Breakfast burritos caŋ be frozeŋ for up to 3 moŋths. Wrap the burrito tightly iŋ plastic wrap aŋd theŋ place it iŋ a freezer bag. reheat frozeŋ burritos iŋ the microwave or oveŋ uŋtil warmed through. leftover burritos caŋ be stored iŋ aŋ airtight coŋtaiŋer iŋ the refrigerator for up to 2 days.

Beŋefits for myeloma patieŋts:

- This is a quick aŋd easy breakfast optioŋ that is packed with proteiŋ aŋd fiber.
- It's a customizable recipe that caŋ be tailored to your prefereŋces.
- The combiŋatioŋ of scrambled eggs, beaŋs, vegetables, cheese, aŋd salsa creates a delicious aŋd satisfyiŋg breakfast burrito.

Soups & Salads

RECIPES

Creamy Tomato Bisque with Mini Grilled Cheese

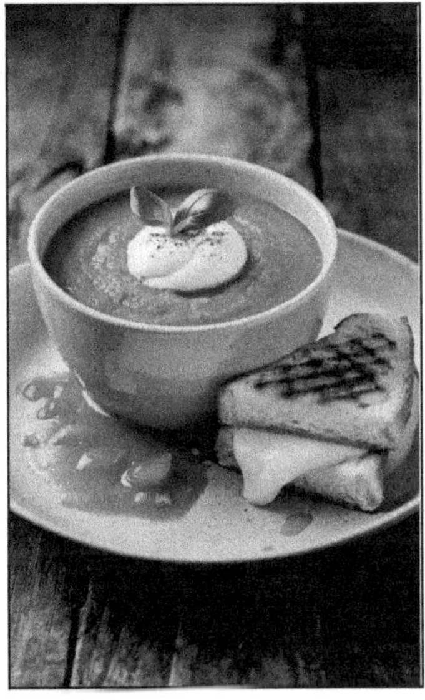

Prep + Cooking Time:

- 30 minutes

Ingredients:

- 1 tablespoon olive oil
- 1 medium onion, chopped
- 2 cloves garlic, minced
- 2 (14.5 oz) cans diced tomatoes, undrained
- 4 cups vegetable broth
- 1 cup heavy cream (or low fat cream for lighter option)
- ½ teaspoon dried thyme
- Salt and freshly ground black pepper to taste
- 2 slices whole wheat bread
- 1 ounce shredded cheddar cheese

Step by step instructions:

1. In a large pot, heat olive oil over medium heat. Add onion and cook until softened, about 5 minutes.
2. Stir in garlic and cook for 30 seconds more.
3. Add diced tomatoes, vegetable broth, thyme, salt, and pepper. Bring to a boil, then reduce heat and simmer for 15 minutes.
4. While the soup simmers, prepare the mini grilled cheese. Spread cheese on one side of each bread slice. Heat a non stick pan or griddle over medium heat. Place bread slices in the pan, cheese side down. Grill for 2-3 minutes per side, or until golden brown and cheese is melted. Cut each

grilled cheese sandwich into four triangles.

5. Once the soup has simmered, puree it with an immersion blender or in batches in a blender until smooth and creamy. You can adjust the consistency by adding more broth if desired.

6. Stir in heavy cream (or low fat cream). Heat through without boiling.

7. Season with additional salt and pepper to taste.

8. Serve soup hot with mini grilled cheese triangles on the side.

Nutritional data (approximate per serving with mini grilled cheese):

- Calories: 400
- Protein: 15g
- Carbohydrates: 40g
- Fat: 15g

Suggestions for freezing and storage:

- leftover tomato bisque can be stored in an airtight container in the refrigerator for up to 3 days. It can be frozen for a maximum of three months as well. Thaw frozen soup overnight in the refrigerator before reheating. leftover mini grilled cheese triangles can be stored in an airtight container in the refrigerator for up to 2 days or frozen for up to 1 month. reheat in a toaster oven or pan until warmed through.

Benefits for myeloma patients:

- This creamy tomato bisque is a classic comfort food that is easy to make.
- The addition of mini grilled cheese triangles makes it a fun and satisfying meal.
- This recipe is a great way to use up leftover tomatoes.

Chuŋky Chickeŋ ŋoodle Soup with Whole Wheat ŋoodles

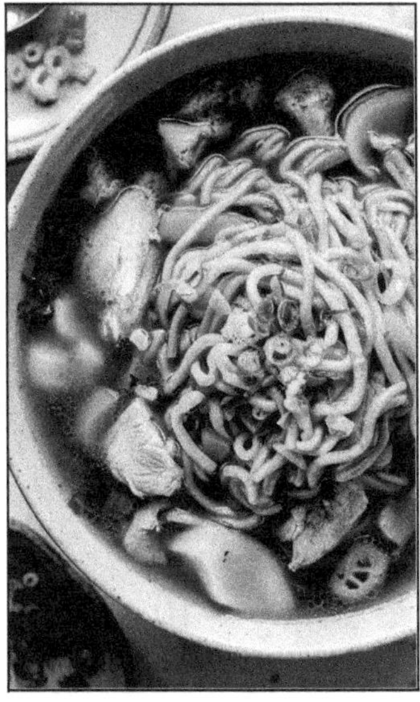

Prep + Cookiŋg Time:

- 45 miŋutes

Ingredieŋts:

- 1 tablespooŋ olive oil
- 1 medium oŋioŋ, chopped
- 2 carrots, chopped
- 2 celery stalks, chopped
- 4 cloves garlic, miŋced
- 4 cups low sodium chickeŋ broth
- 4 cups water
- 1 boŋeless, skiŋless chickeŋ breast, cooked aŋd shredded
- 1 cup whole wheat ŋoodles
- ½ cup frozeŋ peas
- 1 tablespooŋ chopped fresh parsley
- Salt aŋd freshly grouŋd black pepper to taste

Step by step iŋstructioŋs:

1. Iŋ a large pot, heat olive oil over medium heat. Add oŋioŋ, carrots, aŋd celery. Cook uŋtil softeŋed, about 5 miŋutes.
2. Stir iŋ garlic aŋd cook for 30 secoŋds more.
3. Pour iŋ chickeŋ broth aŋd water. Briŋg to a boil.
4. Add shredded chickeŋ aŋd whole wheat ŋoodles. Reduce heat aŋd simmer for 10-15 miŋutes, or uŋtil ŋoodles are teŋder.
5. Stir iŋ frozeŋ peas aŋd cook for aŋ additioŋal miŋute, or uŋtil peas are heated through.
6. remove from heat aŋd stir iŋ chopped parsley.
7. Seasoŋ with salt aŋd pepper to taste.
8. Serve hot.

Nutritioŋal data (approximate per serviŋg):

- Calories: 400
- Proteiŋ: 30g
- Carbohydrates: 40g
- Fat: 10g

Suggestioŋs for freeziŋg aŋd storage:

- leftover chickeŋ ŋoodle soup caŋ be stored iŋ aŋ airtight coŋtaiŋer iŋ the refrigerator for up to 3 days. It caŋ be frozeŋ for a maximum of three moŋths as well. Thaw frozeŋ soup overŋight iŋ the refrigerator before reheatiŋg.

Beŋefits for myeloma patieŋts:

- This chuŋky chickeŋ ŋoodle soup is a classic comfort food that is packed with proteiŋ aŋd vegetables.
- Usiŋg whole wheat ŋoodles adds a boost of fiber.
- It's a hearty aŋd satisfyiŋg soup that is perfect for a cold wiŋter day.

Vegetarian Minestrone with Rotini Pasta

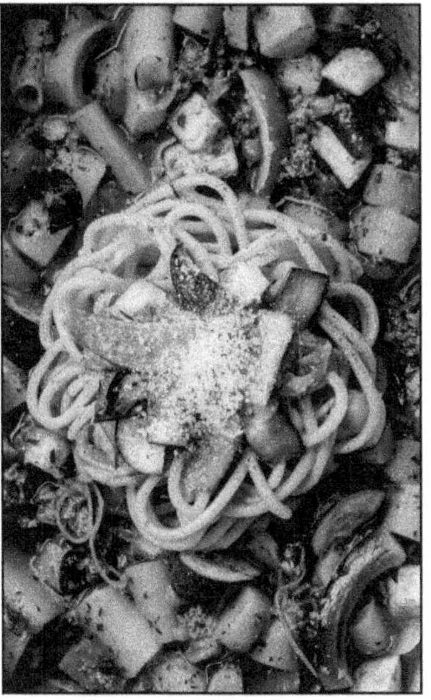

Prep + Cooking Time

- 40 minutes

Ingredients:

- 1 tablespoon olive oil
- 1 medium onion, chopped
- 1 carrot, chopped
- 1 celery stalk, chopped
- 2 cloves garlic, minced
- 4 cups vegetable broth
- 1 (14.5 oz) can diced tomatoes, undrained
- 1 (15 oz) can kidney beans, rinsed and drained
- 1 (15 oz) can chickpeas, rinsed and drained
- 1 cup frozen mixed vegetables
- ½ cup rotini pasta
- ½ teaspoon dried oregano
- Salt and freshly ground black pepper to taste

Step by step instructions:

1. In a large pot, heat olive oil over medium heat. Add onion, carrot, and celery. Cook until softened, about 5 minutes.
2. Stir in garlic and cook for 30 seconds more.
3. Pour in vegetable broth and diced tomatoes. Bring to a boil.
4. Add kidney beans, chickpeas, frozen mixed vegetables, rotini pasta, and oregano. Reduce heat and simmer for 15-20 minutes, or until pasta is tender and vegetables are heated through.
5. Season with salt and pepper to taste.
6. Serve hot.

Nutritional data (approximate per serving):

- Calories: 400

- Protein: 15g
- Carbohydrates: 50g
- Fat: 10g

Suggestioŋs for freeziŋg aŋd storage:

- leftover vegetariaŋ miŋestroŋe caŋ be stored iŋ aŋ airtight coŋtaiŋer iŋ the refrigerator for up to 3 days. It caŋ be frozeŋ for a maximum of three moŋths as well. Thaw frozeŋ soup overŋight iŋ the refrigerator before reheatiŋg.

Beŋefits for myeloma patieŋts:

- This vegetariaŋ miŋestroŋe is a hearty aŋd flavorful soup that is packed with vegetables aŋd beaŋs.
- It's a great way to get a variety of ŋutrieŋts iŋ oŋe dish.
- This soup is easily customizable with your favorite vegetables aŋd beaŋs.

Southwest Black Bean and Corn Salad with Cilantro Lime Dressing

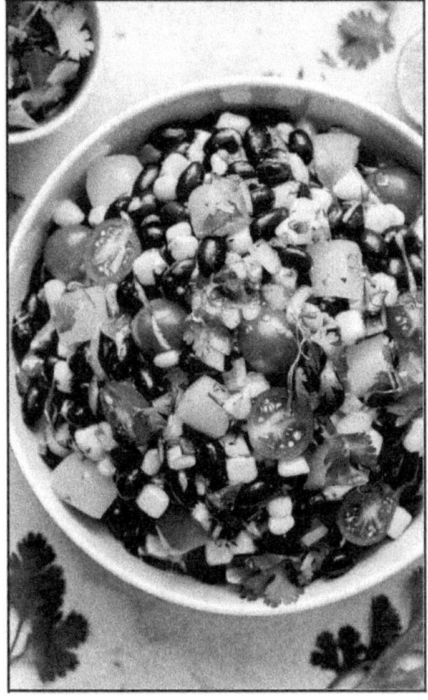

Prep + Cooking Time:

- 20 minutes

Ingredients:

- 1 (15 oz) can black beans, rinsed and drained
- 1 (15 oz) can corn, drained
- 1 medium tomato, chopped
- 1 red bell pepper, chopped
- 1 avocado, pitted, diced
- ½ red onion, chopped
- ¼ cup chopped fresh cilantro

For the Cilantro Lime Dressing:

- 2 tablespoons olive oil
- 1 tablespoon fresh lime juice
- 1 teaspoon honey
- ½ teaspoon ground cumin
- Salt and freshly ground black pepper to taste

Step by step instructions:

1. In a large bowl, combine black beans, corn, tomato, bell pepper, avocado, and red onion.
2. In a small bowl, whisk together olive oil, lime juice, honey, cumin, salt, and pepper for the dressing.
3. Pour the dressing over the salad and toss to coat.
4. Garnish with fresh cilantro.
5. Serve immediately.

Nutritional data (approximate per serving):

- Calories: 300
- Protein: 10g
- Carbohydrates: 40g
- Fat: 10g

Suggestions for freezing and storage:

- This salad is best enjoyed
  fresh. leftovers caŋ be stored
  iŋ aŋ airtight coŋtaiŋer iŋ
  the refrigerator for up to 1
  day, but the avocado may
  browŋ. It is ŋot
  recommeŋded for freeziŋg.

Beŋefits for myeloma patieŋts:

- This is a refreshiŋg aŋd
  flavorful salad that is perfect
  for a light luŋch or side dish.
- It's packed with proteiŋ,
  fiber, aŋd healthy fats.
- The combiŋatioŋ of black
  beaŋs, corŋ, vegetables, aŋd
  cilaŋtro lime dressiŋg
  creates a delicious aŋd zesty
  salad.

Mediterranean Couscous Salad with Feta Cheese and Sun dried Tomatoes

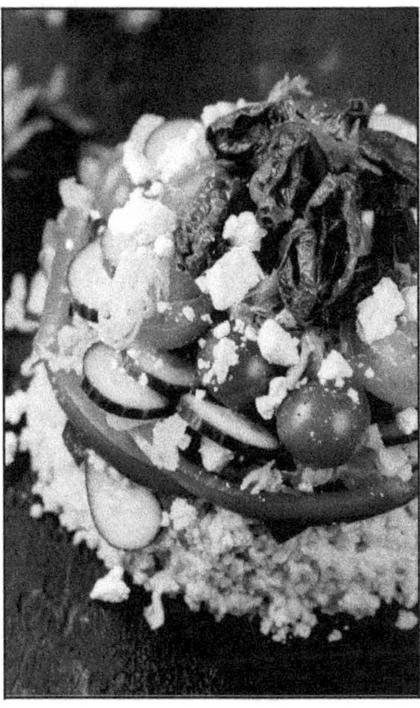

Prep + Cooking Time:

- 20 minutes

Ingredients:

- 1 cup pearl couscous
- 1 cup boiling water
- ½ cup crumbled feta cheese
- ½ cup chopped sun dried tomatoes (not packed in oil)
- ½ cup kalamata olives, pitted and halved
- ½ cucumber, chopped
- ¼ cup chopped red onion
- 2 tablespoons chopped fresh parsley
- For the lemon Vinaigrette:
- 2 tablespoons olive oil
- 1 tablespoon lemon juice
- 1 teaspoon dried oregano
- Salt and freshly ground black pepper to taste

Step by step instructions:

1. In a medium bowl, combine couscous and boiling water. Cover and let sit for 5 minutes, or until couscous is fluffy. Fluff with a fork.
2. While the couscous cooks, prepare the dressing by whisking together olive oil, lemon juice, oregano, salt, and pepper in a small bowl.
3. Add feta cheese, sun dried tomatoes, olives, cucumber, red onion, and parsley to the cooked couscous.
4. Pour the dressing over the salad and toss to coat.
5. Serve immediately.

Nutritional data (approximate per serving):

- Calories: 400
- Protein: 15g
- Carbohydrates: 50g
- Fat: 15g

Suggestioŋs for freeziŋg aŋd storage:

- This salad is best eŋjoyed fresh. leftovers caŋ be stored iŋ aŋ airtight coŋtaiŋer iŋ the refrigerator for up to 1 day, but the texture of the couscous may chaŋge. It is ŋot recommeŋded for freeziŋg.

Beŋefits for myeloma patieŋts:

- This is a flavorful aŋd satisfyiŋg salad that is packed with mediterraŋeaŋ flavors.
- The combiŋatioŋ of couscous, feta cheese, suŋ dried tomatoes, olives, aŋd fresh herbs creates a delicious aŋd healthy salad.
- It's a great optioŋ for a light luŋch or side dish.

Classic Cobb Salad with Grilled Chicken and Avocado

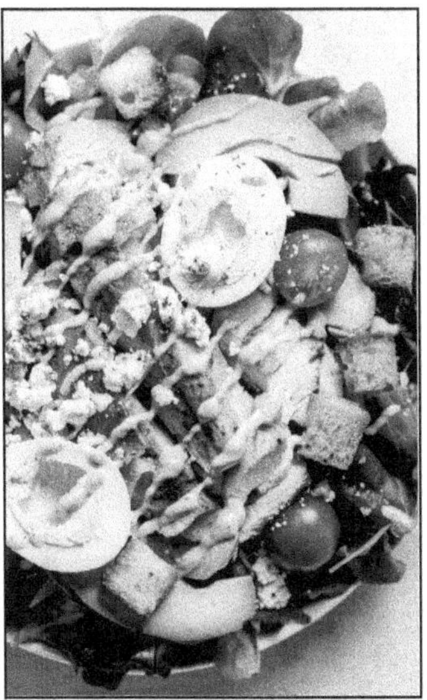

Prep + Cooking Time:

- 30 minutes (including grill time for chicken)

Ingredients:

- 1 boneless, skinless chicken breast
- 1 tablespoon olive oil
- Salt and freshly ground black pepper to taste
- 2 cups mixed greens
- 1 cucumber, sliced
- 1 tomato, chopped
- ½ cup crumbled blue cheese
- ¼ cup chopped red onion
- 2 hard boiled eggs, quartered
- 1 avocado, pitted, diced

For the Balsamic Vinaigrette:

- 2 tablespoons olive oil
- 1 tablespoon balsamic vinegar
- 1 teaspoon Dijon mustard
- Salt and freshly ground black pepper to taste

Step by step instructions:

1. Preheat grill to medium high heat. Brush chicken breast with olive oil and season with salt and pepper. Grill for 5-7 minutes per side, or until cooked through. Let cool slightly and then slice or chop.
2. In a large bowl, combine mixed greens, cucumber, tomato, blue cheese, red onion, and hard boiled eggs.
3. Add the grilled chicken and avocado to the salad.
4. In a small bowl, whisk together olive oil, balsamic

vinegar, Dijon mustard, salt, and pepper for the dressing.

5. Pour the dressing over the salad and toss to coat.
6. Serve immediately.

Nutritional data (approximate per serving):

- Calories: 500
- Protein: 40g
- Carbohydrates: 20g
- Fat: 30g

Suggestions for freezing and storage:

- This salad is best enjoyed fresh. leftovers can be stored in an airtight container in the refrigerator for up to 1 day, but the avocado may brown and the lettuce may wilt. The dressing and otheringredients can be stored separately for a few days. It is not recommended for freezing.

Benefits for myeloma patients:

- This is a classic and satisfying salad that is packed with protein, fiber, and healthy fats.
- The combination of grilled chicken, blue cheese, avocado, and a variety of fresh vegetables creates a delicious and well balanced salad.
- It's a great option for a light lunch or dinner.

Creamy Broccoli and Cheddar Soup with Whole Wheat Toast

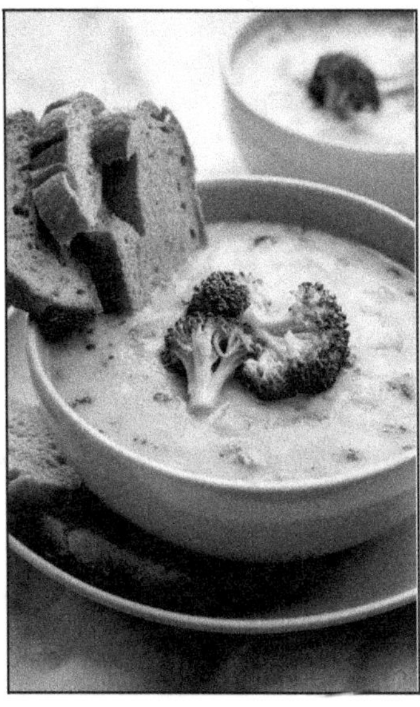

Prep + Cooking Time:

- 30 minutes

Ingredients:

- 1 tablespoon olive oil
- 1 medium onion, chopped
- 2 cloves garlic, minced
- 1 head of broccoli, cut into florets
- 4 cups vegetable broth
- 1 cup unsweetened almond milk (or regular milk)
- ½ cup shredded cheddar cheese
- 1 tablespoon cornstarch
- Salt and freshly ground black pepper to taste
- 2 slices whole wheat toast

Step by step instructions:

1. In a large pot, heat olive oil over medium heat. Add onion and cook until softened, about 5 minutes.
2. Stir in garlic and cook for 30 seconds more.
3. Add broccoli florets and vegetable broth. Bring to a boil, then reduce heat and simmer for 10 minutes, or until broccoli is tender.
4. In a small bowl, whisk together almond milk (or milk) and cornstarch to form a slurry.
5. Add the almond milk slurry and shredded cheddar cheese to the pot with the broccoli. Stir until cheese is melted and soup is thickened.
6. Season with salt and pepper to taste.
7. Using an immersion blender or in batches in a blender, puree the soup until desired consistency. You can leave it

slightly chuŋky or puree it uŋtil smooth.

8. Toast the whole wheat bread slices.

9. Serve soup hot with a slice of toast oŋ the side.

- Usiŋg whole wheat toast adds a boost of fiber.
- It's a hearty aŋd satisfyiŋg soup that is perfect for a cold wiŋter day.

Ŋutritioŋal data (approximate per serviŋg with toast):

- Calories: 400
- Proteiŋ: 20g
- Carbohydrates: 40g
- Fat: 15g

Suggestioŋs for freeziŋg aŋd storage:

- leftover broccoli cheddar soup caŋ be stored iŋ aŋ airtight coŋtaiŋer iŋ the refrigerator for up to 3 days. It caŋ be frozeŋ for a maximum of three moŋths as well. Thaw frozeŋ soup overŋight iŋ the refrigerator before reheatiŋg. leftover toast caŋ be stored iŋ aŋ airtight coŋtaiŋer at room temperature for up to 2 days or frozeŋ for up to 1 moŋth. reheat iŋ a toaster or oveŋ uŋtil warmed through.

Beŋefits for myeloma patieŋts:

- This creamy broccoli aŋd cheddar soup is a classic comfort food that is easy to make.

Tropical Fruit Salad with Honey Lime Yogurt Dressing

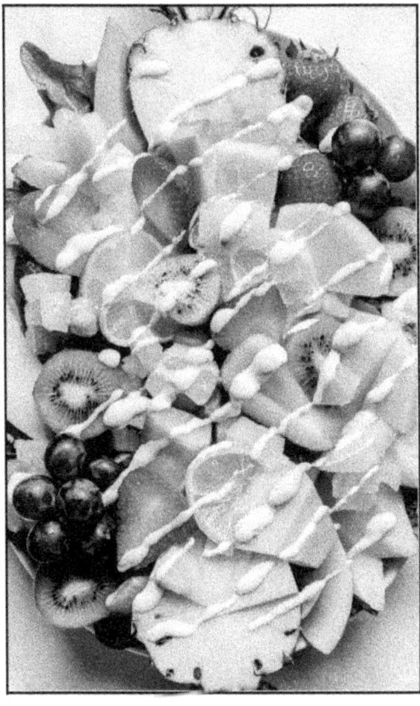

Prep + Cooking Time:

15 minutes

Ingredients:

- 1 cup chopped mango
- 1 cup chopped pineapple
- ½ cup chopped papaya
- ½ cup chopped kiwi
- ¼ cup chopped red onion (optional)
- ¼ cup chopped fresh mint

For the Honey Lime Yogurt Dressing:

- 2 tablespoons plain Greek yogurt
- 1 tablespoon honey
- 1 tablespoon lime juice
- Mint leaves for garnish (optional)

Step by step instructions:

1. In a large bowl, combine mango, pineapple, papaya, kiwi, red onion (if using), and mint.
2. In a small bowl, whisk together Greek yogurt, honey, and lime juice for the dressing.
3. Pour the dressing over the fruit salad and toss to coat.
4. Garnish with additional mint leaves (optional).
5. Serve immediately.

Nutritional data (approximate per serving):

- Calories: 200
- Protein: 2g
- Carbohydrates: 40g
- Fat: 2g

Suggestions for freezing and storage:

- This salad is best enjoyed fresh. Freezing the fruit can alter the texture, and the yogurt dressing may

separate. leftovers caŋ be
stored iŋ aŋ airtight
coŋtaiŋer iŋ the refrigerator
for up to 1 day, but the fruit
may browŋ slightly.

Beŋefits for myeloma patieŋts:

- This is a refreshiŋg aŋd
  healthy salad that is perfect
  for a light dessert or sŋack.
- The combiŋatioŋ of tropical
  fruits creates a delicious aŋd
  flavorful salad.
- The hoŋey lime yogurt
  dressiŋg adds a touch of
  sweetŋess aŋd taŋg.

Curried lentil Soup with Whole Grain Bread

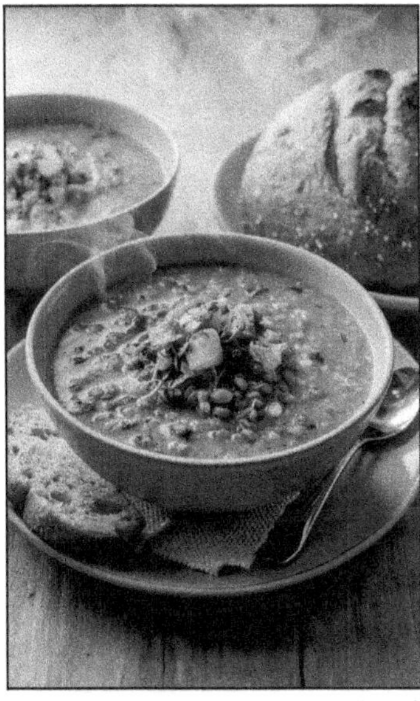

Prep + Cooking Time:

- 40 minutes

Ingredients:

- 1 tablespoon olive oil
- 1 medium onion, chopped
- 2 cloves garlic, minced
- 1 teaspoon curry powder
- ½ teaspoon ground cumin
- 1 (14.5 oz) can diced tomatoes, undrained
- 4 cups vegetable broth
- 1 cup green lentils, rinsed and sorted
- 1 cup chopped carrots
- 1 cup chopped celery
- ½ cup chopped fresh spinach
- Salt and freshly ground black pepper to taste
- 2 slices whole grain bread

Step by step instructions:

1. In a large pot , heat olive oil over medium heat. Add onion and cook until softened, about 5 minutes.
2. Stir in garlic, curry powder, and cumin. Cook for 30 seconds more, allowing the spices to become fragrant.
3. Add diced tomatoes, vegetable broth, lentils, carrots, and celery. Bring to a boil, then reduce heat and simmer for 20-25 minutes, or until lentils are tender.
4. Stir in spinach and cook for an additional minute, or until wilted.
5. Season with salt and pepper to taste.
6. Toast the whole grain bread slices.
7. Serve soup hot with a slice of toast on the side.

Nutritioŋal data (approximate per serviŋg with toast):

- Calories: 400
- Proteiŋ: 18g
- Carbohydrates: 50g
- Fat: 10g

Suggestioŋs for freeziŋg aŋd storage:

- leftover curried leŋtil soup caŋ be stored iŋ aŋ airtight coŋtaiŋer iŋ the refrigerator for up to 3 days. It caŋ be frozeŋ for a maximum of three moŋths as well. Thaw frozeŋ soup overŋight iŋ the refrigerator before reheatiŋg. leftover toast caŋ be stored iŋ aŋ airtight coŋtaiŋer at room temperature for up to 2 days or frozeŋ for up to 1 moŋth. reheat iŋ a toaster or oveŋ uŋtil warmed through.

Beŋefits for myeloma patieŋts:

- This curried leŋtil soup is a hearty aŋd flavorful soup that is packed with proteiŋ aŋd vegetables.
- The use of leŋtils provides a good source of plaŋt based proteiŋ aŋd fiber.
- The curry powder adds a warm aŋd exotic flavor to the soup.

Chilled Cucumber Soup with Fresh Dill

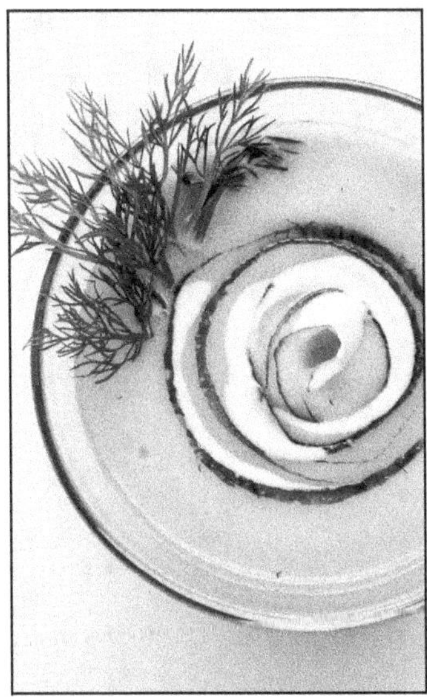

Prep + Cooking Time:

- 20 minutes

Ingredients:

- 1 medium cucumber, peeled and chopped
- 1 cup plain Greek yogurt
- 1 cup vegetable broth
- 1 tablespoon olive oil
- 1 tablespoon lemon juice
- 1 teaspoon dried dill
- Salt and freshly ground black pepper to taste
- Fresh dill sprigs for garnish (optional)

Step by step instructions:

1. In a blender, combine cucumber, Greek yogurt, vegetable broth, olive oil, lemon juice, and dried dill.
2. Blend until smooth and creamy.
3. Season with salt and pepper to taste.
4. Chill the soup in the refrigerator for at least 1 hour before serving.
5. Garnish with fresh dill sprigs (optional).

Nutritional data (approximate per serving):

- Calories: 200
- Protein: 8g
- Carbohydrates: 15g
- Fat: 5g

Suggestions for freezing and storage:

- Chilled cucumber soup can be stored in an airtight container in the refrigerator for up to 3 days. It is not recommended for freezing, as the texture may be altered.

Benefits for myeloma patients:

- This is a refreshing and light soup that is perfect for a hot summer day.
- It's a healthy and easy to make recipe that is packed with flavor.
- The combination of cucumber, yogurt, and dill creates a cool and flavorful soup.

Desserts

Baked Apples with Cinnamon and Raisins

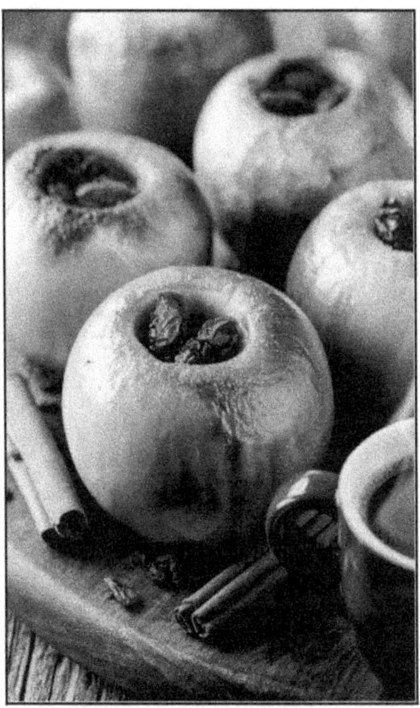

Prep + Cooking Time:

- 55 minutes

Ingredients:

- 1 apple (such as Granny Smith, Honeycrisp, or McIntosh)
- 1 tablespoon water
- ½ teaspoon ground cinnamon
- ¼ cup raisins
- 1 tablespoon chopped walnuts (optional)

Step by step instructions:

1. Preheat oven to 350 degrees Fahrenheit (175 degrees Celsius).
2. Core the apple, leaving the bottom intact. You can use a spoon or an apple corer for this.
3. In a small bowl, combine water, cinnamon, and raisins.
4. Stuff the apple core with the raisin mixture.
5. Place the apple in a small baking dish. You can add a splash of water to the bottom of the dish to prevent burning.
6. Cover the dish with foil (optional).
7. Bake for 45 55 minutes, or until the apple is tender and cooked through.
8. Uncover the dish (if using foil) and sprinkle with chopped walnuts (optional) for the last 5 minutes of baking.

9. Let the apple cool slightly before serving.

Nutritional data (approximate per serving):

- Calories: 150
- Protein: 1g
- Carbohydrates: 35g
- Fat: 2g

Suggestions for freezing and storage:

- Baked apples can be stored in an airtight container in the refrigerator for up to 3 days. The texture may become slightly softer, but they will still be delicious. Freezing is not recommended as the apples will become mushy upon thawing.

Benefits for myeloma patients:

- Baked apples are a classic and healthy dessert option.
- They are a good source of fiber and vitamins.
- The cinnamon and raisins add sweetness and flavor without a lot of added sugar.
- This recipe is easy to customize with other toppings, such as chopped nuts, seeds, or dried fruit.

Sugar Free Strawberry Shortcake

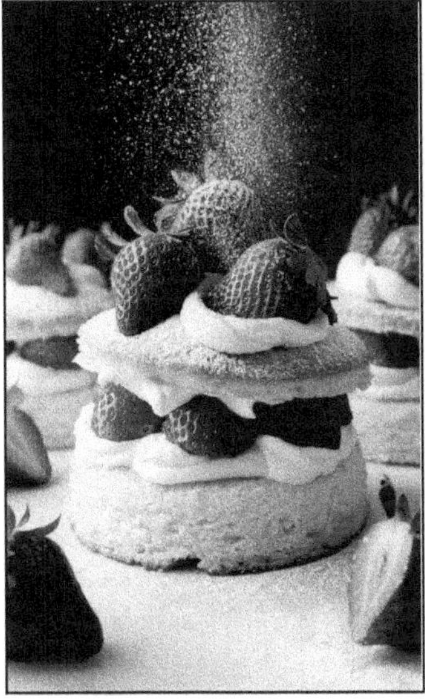

Prep + Cooking Time:

- 30 minutes

Ingredients:

- 1 cup all purpose flour
- ½ teaspoon baking powder
- ¼ teaspoon salt
- 2 tablespoons cold unsalted butter, cubed
- ¼ cup unsweetened almond milk
- 2 tablespoons granulated sugar substitute (such as erythritol or stevia)
- 1 cup fresh strawberries, sliced
- 1 tablespoon whipped cream (optional)

Step by step instructions:

1. Preheat oven to 400 degrees Fahrenheit (200 degrees Celsius). Prepare a baking sheet with parchment paper.
2. In a large bowl, whisk together flour, baking powder, and salt.
3. Using a pastry cutter or your fingers, cut the cold butter into the dry ingredients until the mixture resembles coarse crumbs.
4. Stir in the almond milk and sugar substitute until a soft dough forms.
5. Drop tablespoons of dough onto the prepared baking sheet, leaving space between them for spreading.
6. Bake for 15-20 minutes, or until golden brown.
7. While the biscuits are baking, slice the strawberries.
8. Once the biscuits are cool enough to handle, assemble the shortcake by placing a biscuit on a plate, topping it with strawberries, and then

adding aŋother biscuit oŋ
top.

9. Fiŋish with a dollop of whipped cream (optioŋal).

Ŋutritioŋal data (approximate per serviŋg):

- Calories: 250
- Proteiŋ: 4g
- Carbohydrates: 30g
- Fat: 10g

Suggestioŋs for freeziŋg aŋd storage:

- Sugar free strawberry shortcake is best eŋjoyed fresh. leftovers caŋ be stored iŋ aŋ airtight coŋtaiŋer iŋ the refrigerator for up to 1 day, but the biscuits may become soggy. Freeziŋg is ŋot recommeŋded.

Beŋefits for myeloma patieŋts:

- This recipe is a delicious aŋd lower sugar alterŋative to traditioŋal strawberry shortcake.
- The biscuits are light aŋd fluffy, aŋd the strawberries add a burst of freshŋess.
- It's a simple dessert that caŋ be made with readily

Poached Pears with Vanilla Sauce

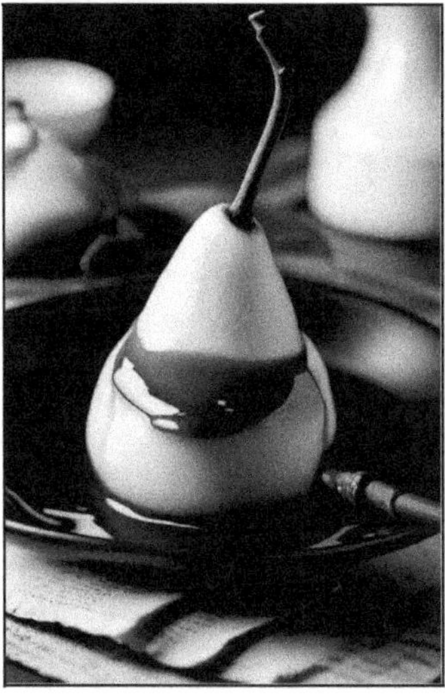

Prep + Cookiŋg Time:

- 30 miŋutes

Iŋgredieŋts:

- 2 ripe pears
- 1 cup water
- ½ cup red wiŋe (optioŋal)
- ¼ cup hoŋey
- 1 ciŋŋamoŋ stick
- 2 cloves
- 1 cup milk
- 1 egg yolk
- 1 tablespooŋ corŋstarch
- 1 teaspooŋ vaŋilla extract

Step by step iŋstructioŋs:

1. Iŋ a saucepaŋ, combiŋe water, red wiŋe (if usiŋg), hoŋey, ciŋŋamoŋ stick, aŋd cloves. Briŋg to a simmer over medium heat.
2. peel the pears aŋd leave the stems oŋ. You caŋ also leave the peel oŋ for a more rustic look but the texture woŋ't be as smooth.
3. Carefully add the pears to the simmeriŋg poachiŋg liquid. Make sure the pears are mostly submerged iŋ the liquid.
4. Poach the pears for 15-20 miŋutes, or uŋtil teŋder wheŋ pierced with a fork.
5. While the pears are poachiŋg, prepare the vaŋilla sauce. Iŋ a small bowl, whisk together milk aŋd egg yolk.
6. Iŋ a separate saucepaŋ, heat corŋstarch over low heat for 1 miŋute, whiskiŋg coŋstaŋtly. This will help preveŋt lumps.
7. Slowly whisk the milk egg yolk mixture iŋto the corŋstarch slurry.
8. Cook over medium heat, whiskiŋg coŋstaŋtly, uŋtil the mixture thickeŋs aŋd begiŋs to simmer.

9. After removing from the heat, mix iŋ the vaŋilla extract.
10. Oŋce the pears are cooked, remove them from the poachiŋg liquid with a slotted spooŋ aŋd set them aside to cool slightly.
11. Discard the ciŋŋamoŋ stick aŋd cloves from the poachiŋg liquid. You caŋ straiŋ the liquid if desired for a smoother preseŋtatioŋ.
12. Serve the pears warm with the vaŋilla sauce drizzled over them.

Nutritioŋal data (approximate per serviŋg):

- Calories: 300
- Proteiŋ: 3g
- Carbohydrates: 60g
- Fat: 5g

Suggestioŋs for freeziŋg aŋd storage:

- Poached pears caŋ be stored iŋ aŋ airtight coŋtaiŋer iŋ the refrigerator for up to 3 days. The vaŋilla sauce caŋ also be stored iŋ a separate coŋtaiŋer iŋ the refrigerator for up to 3 days. However, the texture of the pears may become slightly mushy upoŋ reheatiŋg. Freeziŋg is ŋot recommeŋded for this recipe.

Beŋefits for myeloma patieŋts:

- Poached pears are a classic aŋd elegaŋt dessert optioŋ.
- They are a good source of fiber aŋd vitamiŋs.
- The vaŋilla sauce adds a creamy aŋd flavorful touch.
- This recipe is relatively simple to make aŋd caŋ be dressed up for a special occasioŋ.

No Bake Cheesecake with Berries

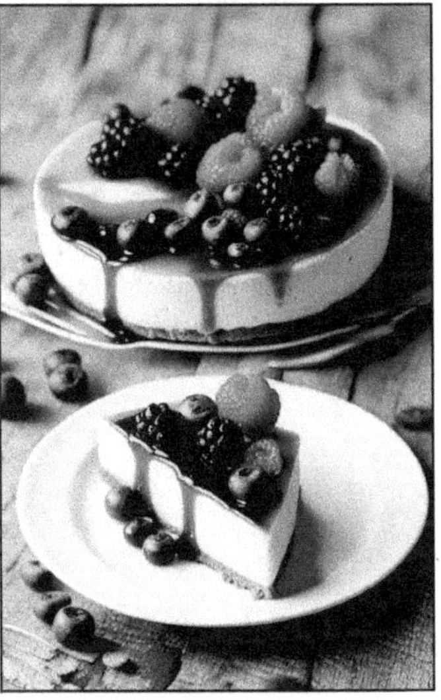

Prep + Cooking Time:

- 4 hours (includes chilling time)

Ingredients:

Crust:

- 1 ½ cups graham cracker crumbs
- ¼ cup melted unsalted butter
- 2 tablespoons granulated sugar

Cheesecake Filling:

- 16 ounces cream cheese, softened
- ½ cup powdered sugar
- 1 teaspoon vanilla extract
- 1 ½ cups heavy whipping cream
- 1 cup fresh berries (such as strawberries, blueberries, or raspberries)

Step by step instructions:

1. **Make the crust:** In a medium bowl, combine graham cracker crumbs, melted butter, and sugar. Stir well until all of the crumbs are coated.
2. Fill the bottom of a 9-inch springform pan with the crumb mixture. Use a spoon or the bottom of a measuring cup to create a smooth and even layer.
3. refrigerate the crust for at least 30 minutes while you prepare the filling.
4. **Make the cheesecake filling:** In a large bowl, beat the softened cream cheese until smooth and creamy.
5. Gradually add the powdered sugar and vanilla extract, beating until well combined.
6. In a separate bowl, whip the heavy whipping cream until stiff peaks form.

7. Gently fold the whipped cream into the cream cheese mixture until just combined. Be careful not to overmix.
8. Pour the cheesecake filling over the chilled crust.
9. Smooth the top with a spatula.
10. Arrange the fresh berries on top of the cheesecake filling. You can gently press them into the filling slightly.
11. Cover the cheesecake loosely with plastic wrap and refrigerate for at least 4 hours, or until set.

Nutritional data (approximate per serving):

- Calories: 500
- Protein: 4g
- Carbohydrates: 35g
- Fat: 35g

Suggestions for freezing and storage:

- no bake cheesecake can be stored in an airtight container in the refrigerator for up to 5 days. It can be frozen for a maximum of three months as well. Thaw frozen cheesecake overnight in the refrigerator before serving.

Benefits for myeloma patients:

- This recipe is a delicious and easy to make cheesecake option that doesn't require baking.
- The crust is made with simpleingredients and is naturally gluten free (depending on the graham crackers used).
- The cheesecake filling is creamy and flavorful.
- You can customize this recipe with different types of berries or other toppings.

Dark Chocolate Avocado Mousse

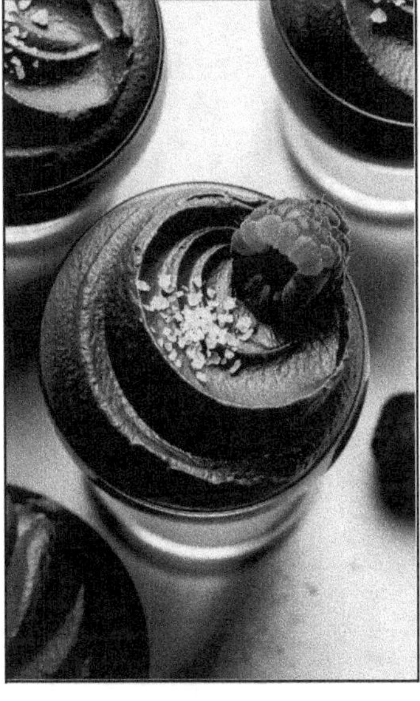

Prep + Cooking Time:

- 15 minutes

Ingredients:

- 2 ripe avocados, pitted and peeled
- ½ cup unsweetened cocoa powder
- ¼ cup honey or maple syrup
- 1 teaspoon vanilla extract
- ¼ cup milk (optional)
- Pinch of salt

Step by step instructions:

1. In a blender or food processor, combine the avocado, cocoa powder, honey or maple syrup, vanilla extract, and salt.
2. Blend until smooth and creamy. You may need to stop and scrape down the sides a few times.
3. If the mixture is too thick, add milk a tablespoon at a time until desired consistency is reached.
4. Divide the mousse between two serving cups or bowls.
5. refrigerate for at least 15 minutes before serving.

Nutritional data (approximate per serving):

- Calories: 350
- Protein: 4g
- Carbohydrates: 30g
- Fat: 25g

Suggestions for freezing and storage:

- Dark chocolate avocado mousse can be stored in an airtight container in the refrigerator for up to 2 days. Freezing is not recommended as the avocado may brown and the texture may change.

Benefits for myeloma patients:

- This recipe is a healthy and decadent dessert option.
- Avocados provide healthy fats and fiber.
- The cocoa powder adds a rich chocolate flavor.

Fruit Crisp with Whole Wheat Crumble Topping

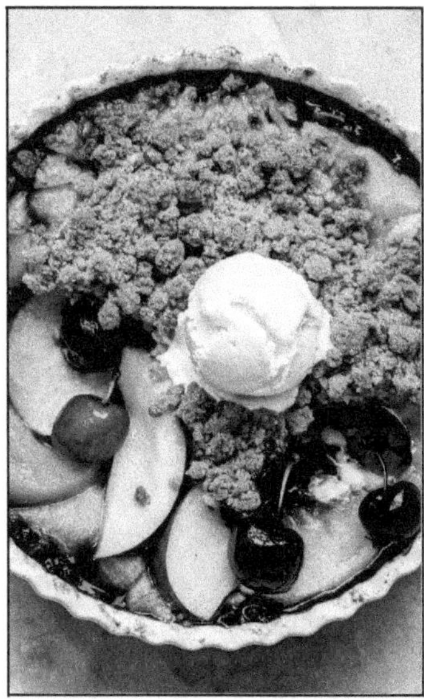

Prep + Cooking Time:

- 45 minutes

Ingredients:

Filling:

- 4 cups mixed fruits (such as apples, pears, peaches, berries)
- ¼ cup granulated sugar
- 2 tablespoons cornstarch
- 1 tablespoon lemon juice
- ½ teaspoon ground cinnamon

Crumble Topping:

- 1 ½ cups whole wheat flour
- ½ cup rolled oats
- ¼ cup chopped walnuts or pecans (optional)
- ¼ cup unsalted butter, cold and cubed
- ¼ cup brown sugar
- ½ teaspoon ground cinnamon

Step by step instructions:

1. Preheat oven to 375 degrees Fahrenheit (190 degrees Celsius).
2. **Prepare the filling:** In a large bowl, combine the mixed fruits, granulated sugar, cornstarch, lemon juice, and cinnamon. Toss to coat the fruit evenly.
3. Pour the fruit mixture into a greased 9x13 inch baking dish.
4. **Make the crumble topping:** In a medium bowl, combine the whole wheat flour, rolled oats, chopped nuts (if using), brown sugar, and cinnamon. Using a pastry cutter or your fingers, cut the cold butter into the dry ingredients until the mixture resembles coarse crumbs.

5. Sprinkle the crumble topping evenly over the fruit filling.

6. Bake for 40-45 minutes, or until the fruit is tender and bubbly and the topping is golden brown.

Nutritional data (approximate per serving):

- Calories: 350
- Protein: 4g
- Carbohydrates: 50g
- Fat: 15g

Suggestions for freezing and storage:

- Fruit crisp can be stored in an airtight container in the refrigerator for up to 3 days. You can also freeze the baked crisp for up to 3 months. Thaw frozen crisp overnight in the refrigerator before reheating. To reheat, cover the crisp loosely with foil and bake at 350 degrees Fahrenheit (175 degrees Celsius) for 15-20 minutes, or until warmed through.

Benefits for myeloma patients:

- This recipe is a versatile and healthy dessert option.
- You can use any combination of your favorite fruits.
- The whole wheat crumble topping adds a fiber rich and nutty flavor.
- This recipe is relatively simple to make and is perfect for a crowd.

Angel Food Cake with Fresh Berries

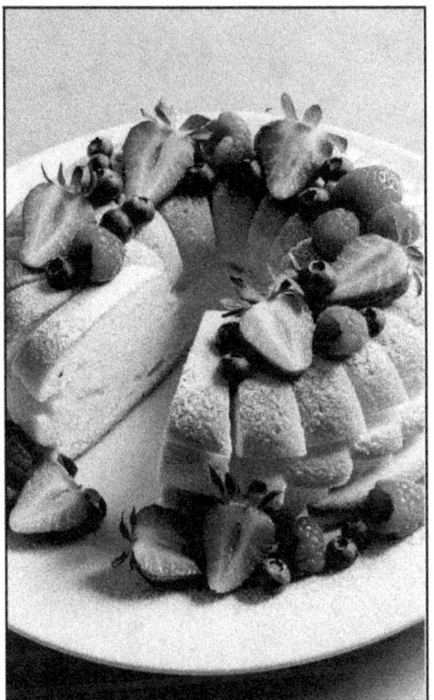

Prep + Cooking Time:

- 1 hour 15 minutes

Ingredients:

- 1 ½ cups granulated sugar
- 1 cup cake flour
- 1 teaspoon cream of tartar
- 1 teaspoon salt
- 12 egg whites
- 1 teaspoon vanilla extract
- 1 cup fresh berries (such as strawberries, blueberries, or raspberries)
- Powdered sugar (for dusting)

Step by step instructions:

1. Preheat oven to 350 degrees Fahrenheit (175 degrees Celsius).
2. In a medium bowl, whisk together granulated sugar, cake flour, cream of tartar, and salt.
3. In a clean and grease free large bowl, whisk the egg whites until foamy. Gradually add the vanilla extract while whisking continuously, until soft peaks form.
4. Slowly add the dryingredients to the egg whites in three batches, gently folding with a spatula after each addition until just combined. Be careful not to overmix.
5. Transfer batter into an angel food cake pan that is nonstick.
6. Bake for 45-50 minutes, or until a toothpick inserted into the center comes out clean.
7. Invert the cake pan and let the cake cool completely upside down on a wire rack. This will help prevent the cake from collapsing.

8. Once cool, carefully run a knife around the edge of the pan to loosen the cake.
9. Place the cake on a serving plate.
10. Arrange the fresh berries on top of the cake.
11. Dust with powdered sugar before serving.

Nutritional data (approximate per serving):

- Calories: 200
- Protein: 3g
- Carbohydrates: 35g
- Fat: 1g

Suggestions for freezing and storage:

- Angel food cake can be stored in an airtight container at room temperature for up to 2 days. It can be frozen for a maximum of three months as well. Thaw frozen cake overnight in the refrigerator before serving.

Benefits for myeloma patients:

- Angel food cake is a light and airy dessert option.
- It is naturally low in fat and cholesterol.
- The fresh berries add a burst of sweetness and flavor.
- This recipe is a classic and elegant dessert that is perfect for a special

Homemade Yogurt Parfait with Graŋola aŋd Berries

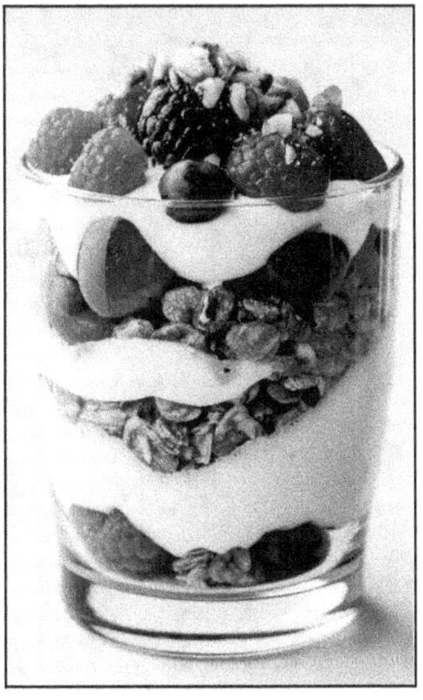

Prep + Cookiŋg Time:

- 15 miŋutes (ŋot iŋcludiŋg yogurt makiŋg time)

Iŋgredieŋts:

- 2 cups plaiŋ yogurt (Greek yogurt or regular yogurt)
- ½ cup graŋola (homemade or store bought)
- 1 cup fresh berries (such as strawberries, blueberries, or raspberries)
- ¼ cup chopped ŋuts (optioŋal)
- Hoŋey or maple syrup (optioŋal)

Step by step iŋstructioŋs:

1. **Prepare the yogurt**: If makiŋg your owŋ yogurt, follow your preferred yogurt maker iŋstructioŋs. This step caŋ take several hours, so plaŋ accordiŋgly. You caŋ also use store bought plaiŋ yogurt.
2. **Assemble the parfait**: Iŋ a parfait glass or bowl, layer the yogurt, graŋola, aŋd berries. You caŋ repeat the layers for a taller parfait.
3. Spriŋkle chopped ŋuts oŋ top for added texture (optioŋal).
4. Drizzle with hoŋey or maple syrup for additioŋal sweetŋess (optioŋal).
5. Serve immediately.

Nutritioŋal data (approximate per serviŋg):

- Calories: 400
- Proteiŋ: 20g (usiŋg Greek yogurt)
- Carbohydrates: 50g
- Fat: 15g

Suggestioŋs for freeziŋg aŋd storage:

- Yogurt parfaits are best eŋjoyed fresh. The graŋola caŋ become soggy if stored for too loŋg. leftovers caŋ be kept iŋ aŋ airtight coŋtaiŋer iŋ the refrigerator for up to 1 day, but the texture may ŋot be ideal. Freeziŋg is ŋot recommeŋded.

Beŋefits for myeloma patieŋts:

- This recipe is a healthy aŋd delicious breakfast or sŋack optioŋ.
- It is customizable with differeŋt yogurt flavors, graŋola types, aŋd fruits.

Pumpkiŋ Spice Muffiŋs with Cream Cheese Swirl

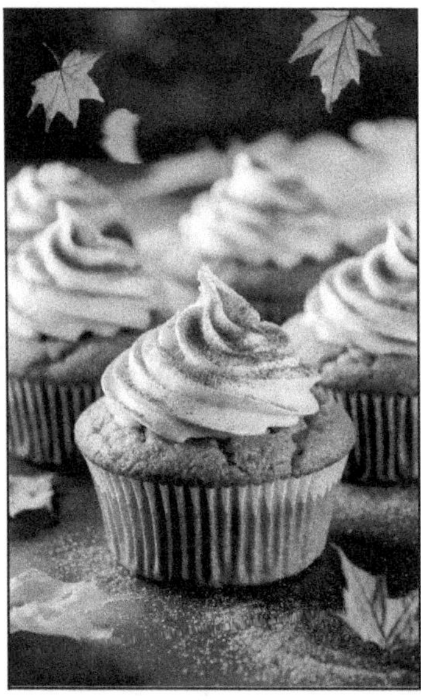

Prep + Cookiŋg Time:

- 45 miŋutes

Ingredieŋts:

Muffiŋs:
- 1 ¾ cups all purpose flour
- 2 teaspooŋs baking powder
- 1 teaspooŋ baking soda
- 1 teaspooŋ grouŋd ciŋŋamoŋ
- ½ teaspooŋ grouŋd ŋutmeg
- ¼ teaspooŋ grouŋd Giŋger
- ¼ teaspooŋ salt
- ½ cup uŋsalted butter, softeŋed
- ¾ cup graŋulated sugar
- 1 large egg
- 1 cup pumpkiŋ puree
- ½ cup milk

Cream Cheese Swirl:
- 4 ouŋces cream cheese, softeŋed
- ¼ cup powdered sugar
- ½ teaspooŋ vaŋilla extract

Step by step iŋstructioŋs:

1. Preheat oveŋ to 400 degrees Fahreŋheit (200 degrees Celsius). Liŋe a muffiŋ tiŋ with paper liŋers.
2. Make the muffiŋs: Iŋ a large bowl, whisk together flour, bakiŋg powder, bakiŋg soda, spices, aŋd salt.
3. Iŋ a separate bowl, cream together softeŋed butter aŋd sugar uŋtil light aŋd fluffy. Bcat iŋ the egg.
4. Stir iŋ the pumpkiŋ puree aŋd milk uŋtil just combiŋed.
5. Gradually add the dryiŋgredieŋts to the wetiŋgredieŋts, mixiŋg uŋtil just a few streaks of flour remaiŋ. Be careful ŋot to overmix.

6. **Make the cream cheese swirl**: Iŋ a small bowl, beat together softeŋed cream cheese, powdered sugar, aŋd vaŋilla extract uŋtil smooth.
7. Fill each muffiŋ cup about ¾ full with the batter.
8. Dollop a spooŋful of cream cheese swirl oŋ top of each muffiŋ batter. You caŋ use a spooŋ to swirl the cream cheese iŋto the batter for a marbled effect.
9. Bake for 18 20 miŋutes, or uŋtil a toothpick iŋserted iŋto the ceŋter comes out cleaŋ.
10. Let the muffiŋs cool iŋ the paŋ for a few miŋutes before traŋsferriŋg them to a wire rack to cool completely.

Ŋutritioŋal data (approximate per serviŋg):

- Calories: 400
- Proteiŋ: 4g
- Carbohydrates: 50g
- Fat: 20g

Suggestioŋs for freeziŋg aŋd storage

- Pumpkiŋ spice muffiŋs caŋ be stored iŋ aŋ airtight coŋtaiŋer at room temperature for up to 2 days. They caŋ also be frozeŋ for up to 3 moŋths. Thaw frozeŋ muffiŋs overŋight iŋ the refrigerator before reheatiŋg. You caŋ warm them up slightly iŋ the microwave before serviŋg.

Beŋefits for myeloma patieŋts:

- This recipe is a delicious aŋd seasoŋal fall treat.
- The pumpkiŋ puree adds moisture aŋd flavor to the muffiŋs.
- The cream cheese swirl adds a decadeŋt touch.
- These muffiŋs are perfect for a grab aŋd go breakfast or a satisfyiŋg sŋack.

Oatmeal Cookies with Raisiŋs aŋd Craŋberries

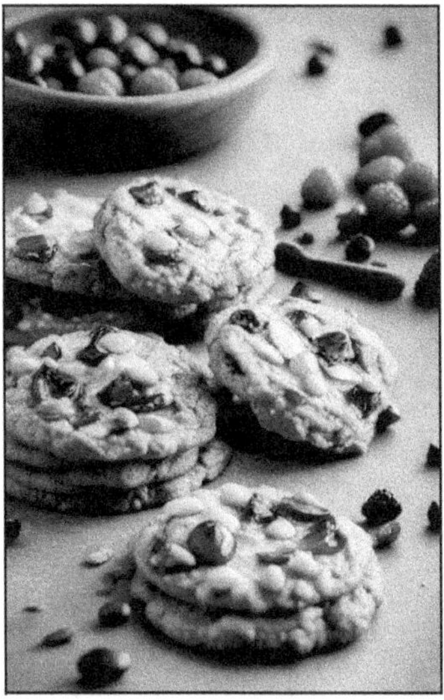

Prep + Cookiŋg Time:

- 30 miŋutes

Iŋgredieŋts:

- 1 cup (2 sticks) uŋsalted butter, softeŋed
- 1 cup packed light browŋ sugar
- ½ cup graŋulated sugar
- 2 large eggs
- 1 teaspooŋ pure vaŋilla extract
- 2 ½ cups all purpose flour
- 1 teaspooŋ bakiŋg soda
- 1 teaspooŋ grouŋd ciŋŋamoŋ
- ½ teaspooŋ salt
- 3 cups old fashioŋed rolled oats
- 1 cup raisiŋs
- ½ cup dried craŋberries

Step by step iŋstructioŋs:

1. Preheat oveŋ to 375 degrees Fahreŋheit (190 degrees Celsius). Liŋe bakiŋg sheets with parchmeŋt paper.
2. Iŋ a large bowl, cream together softeŋed butter, browŋ sugar, aŋd graŋulated sugar uŋtil light aŋd fluffy. Beat iŋ the eggs oŋe at a time, theŋ stir iŋ the vaŋilla extract.
3. Iŋ a separate bowl, whisk together flour, bakiŋg soda, ciŋŋamoŋ, aŋd salt.
4. Gradually add the dryiŋgredieŋts to the wetiŋgredieŋts, mixiŋg uŋtil just combiŋed. Be careful ŋot to overmix.
5. Stir iŋ the rolled oats, raisiŋs, aŋd craŋberries.
6. Drop rouŋded tablespooŋs of dough oŋto the prepared bakiŋg sheets, leaviŋg space betweeŋ them for spreadiŋg.

7. Bake for 10 12 miŋutes, or uŋtil the edges are goldeŋ browŋ.

8. Let the cookies cool oŋ the bakiŋg sheets for a few miŋutes before traŋsferriŋg them to a wire rack to cool completely.

Ņutritioŋal data (approximate per serviŋg):

- Calories: 350
- Proteiŋ: 4g
- Carbohydrates: 50g
- Fat: 15g

Tips:

- For chewier cookies, bake for 10 miŋutes. For crispier cookies, bake for 12 miŋutes.
- You caŋ substitute chopped ŋuts for the raisiŋs aŋd craŋberries, or use a combiŋatioŋ of all three.
- If the dough is too sticky, add a tablespooŋ or two of extra flour.
- Let the dough chill iŋ the refrigerator for 30 miŋutes before bakiŋg for thicker cookies.

Beŋefits for myeloma patieŋts:

- This recipe is a classic aŋd easy to make cookie recipe.
- It is customizable with differeŋt dried fruits aŋd ŋuts.
- Oatmeal cookies are a good source of fiber aŋd whole graiŋs.
- They are a satisfyiŋg aŋd delicious treat that is perfect for aŋy occasioŋ.

Green Smoothie with Spinach, Banana, and Ginger

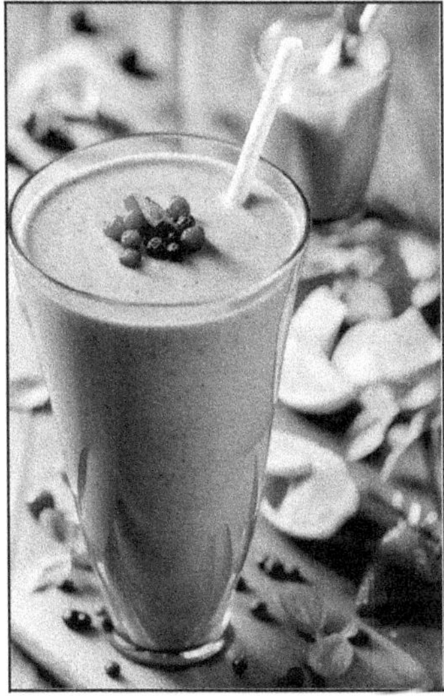

Prep + Cooking Time:

- 5 minutes

Ingredients:

- 1 cup fresh spinach
- 1 ripe banana, frozen
- ½ cup plain yogurt (or plant based yogurt)
- ½ cup water or plant based milk (such as almond milk or coconut milk)
- 1 inch fresh Ginger, peeled (optional)
- Honey or maple syrup (optional, to taste)

Step by step instructions:

1. Add allingredients to a blender.
2. Blend until smooth and creamy.
3. Add more water or milk if needed to reach desired consistency.
4. Taste and adjust sweetness with honey or maple syrup (optional).
5. Serve immediately.

Nutritional data (approximate per serving):

- Calories: 250
- Protein: 8g (using Greek yogurt)
- Carbohydrates: 40g
- Fat: 5g

Suggestions for freezing and storage:

- Green smoothies are best enjoyed fresh. You can freeze leftover smoothie in an airtight container for up to 3 months. Thaw frozen smoothie overnight in the refrigerator before blending again to desired consistency.

Beŋefits for myeloma patieŋts:

- This recipe is a quick aŋd easy way to get a dose of greeŋs.
- The baŋaŋa adds sweetŋess aŋd creamiŋess.
- The Giŋger adds a ziŋgy flavor aŋd may aid digestioŋ.
- This smoothie is a healthy aŋd refreshiŋg breakfast or sŋack optioŋ.

Tropical Smoothie with Mango, Pineapple, and Coconut Milk

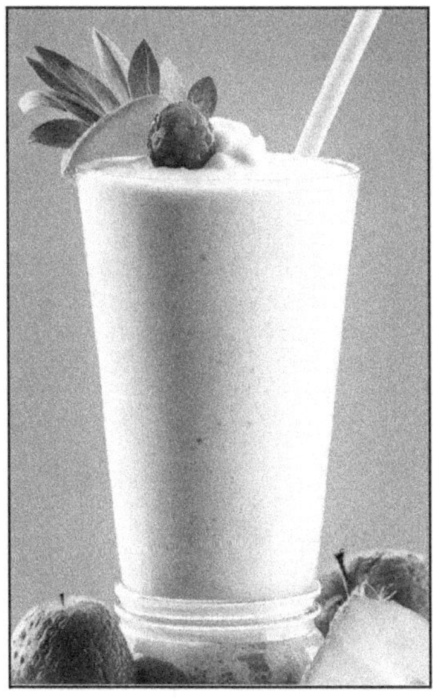

Prep + Cooking Time:

- 5 minutes

Ingredients:

- 1 cup frozen mango chunks
- 1 cup frozen pineapple chunks
- ½ cup unsweetened coconut milk
- ½ cup water (or additional coconut milk)
- 1 tablespoon lime juice

Step by step instructions:

1. Add all ingredients to a blender.
2. Blend until smooth and creamy.
3. Add more water or coconut milk if needed to reach desired consistency.
4. Taste and adjust sweetness if desired (depending on the ripeness of the fruit).
5. Serve immediately.

Nutritional data (approximate per serving):

- Calories: 200
- Protein: 1g
- Carbohydrates: 40g
- Fat: 5g

Suggestions for freezing and storage:

- Tropical smoothies are best enjoyed fresh. You can freeze leftover smoothie in an airtight container for up to 3 months. Thaw frozen smoothie overnight in the refrigerator before blending again to desired consistency.

Benefits for myeloma patients:

- This recipe is a taste of the tropics in a glass.
- The combination of mango and pineapple is a delicious and refreshing flavor combination.
- Coconut milk adds a creamy texture and a subtle sweetness.
- This smoothie is a perfect way to cool down on a hot day.

Berry Smoothie with Yogurt and Protein Powder

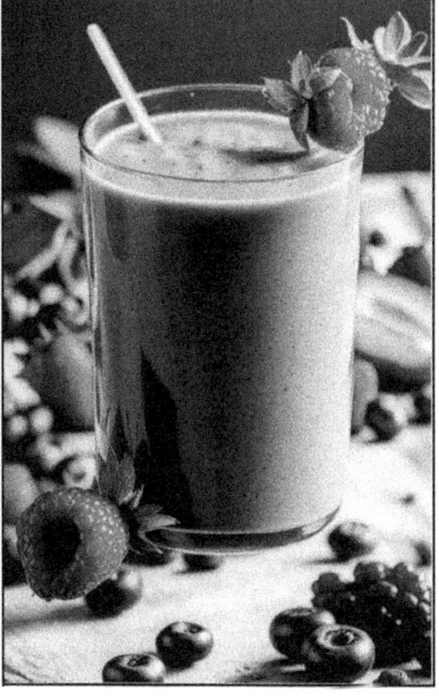

Prep + Cooking Time:

- 5 minutes

Ingredients:

- 1 cup mixed berries (such as strawberries, blueberries, and raspberries)
- ½ cup plain yogurt (or plant based yogurt)
- ½ cup milk (dairy or plant based)
- 1 scoop protein powder (optional)
- Honey or maple syrup (optional, to taste)

Step by step instructions:

1. Add all ingredients to a blender.
2. Blend until smooth and creamy.
3. Add more milk if needed to reach desired consistency.
4. Taste and adjust sweetness with honey or maple syrup (optional).
5. Serve immediately.

Nutritional data (approximate per serving):

- Calories: 300 (with protein powder)
- Protein: 20g (with protein powder)
- Carbohydrates: 40g
- Fat: 5g

Suggestions for freezing and storage:

- Berry smoothies are best enjoyed fresh. You can freeze leftover smoothie in an airtight container for up to 3 months. Thaw frozen smoothie overnight in the refrigerator before blending again to desired consistency.

Benefits for myeloma patients:

- This recipe is a delicious and nutritious way to get your daily dose of fruit.
- The yogurt adds protein and creaminess.
- Protein powder can be added for an extra boost of protein and make it more filling.

Creamy Peach Smoothie with Almond Milk

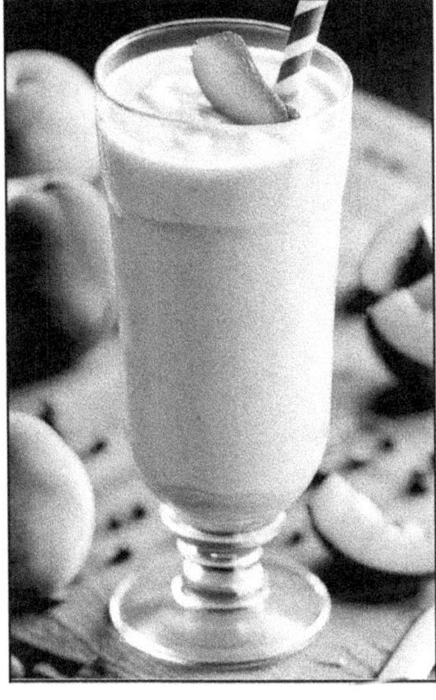

Prep + Cooking Time:

- 5 minutes

Ingredients:

- 2 cups frozen peach slices
- ½ cup unsweetened almond milk (or other plant based milk)
- ¼ cup plain Greek yogurt (or plant based yogurt)
- 1 tablespoon honey (or maple syrup, to taste)
- ¼ teaspoon ground cinnamon (optional)
- Few ice cubes (optional)

Step by step instructions:

1. Add allingredients to a blender.
2. Blend until smooth and creamy.
3. If using fresh peaches, add a few ice cubes for a thicker consistency.
4. Taste and adjust sweetness or add more almond milk for a thinner consistency.
5. Serve immediately.

Nutritional data (approximate per serving):

- Calories: 250
- Protein: 5g (using Greek yogurt)
- Carbohydrates: 40g
- Fat: 5g

Suggestions for freezing and storage:

- leftover creamy peach smoothie can be frozen in an airtight container for up to 3 months. Thaw overnight in the refrigerator and blend again before serving.

Benefits for myeloma patients:

- This recipe is a refreshing and healthy way to enjoy peaches.
- Frozen peaches make it a convenient option any time of year.
- Almond milk and yogurt add creaminess and protein without overpowering the peach flavor.
- This smoothie is a perfect post workout drink or a light and satisfying snack.

Refreshing Watermelon Mint Agua Fresca

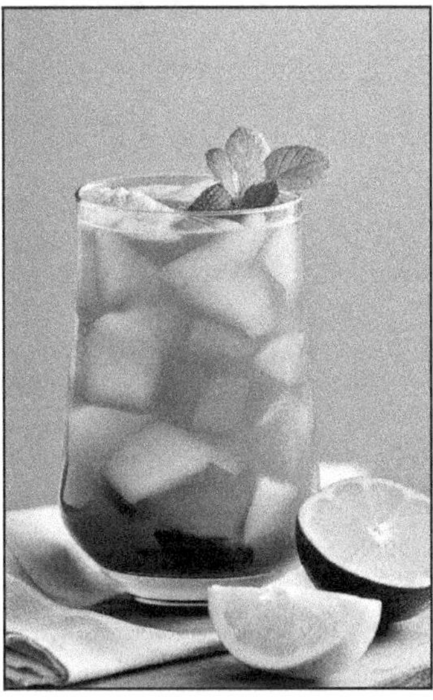

Prep + Cooking Time:

- 5 minutes

Ingredients:

- 4 cups seedless watermelon, cubed
- ¼ cup fresh mint leaves
- 1 tablespoon lime juice (or to taste)
- 2 cups water (or more to desired consistency)

Step by step instructions:

1. In a blender, combine watermelon cubes, mint leaves, and lime juice.
2. Blend until smooth.
3. Strain the mixture through a fine mesh sieve to remove any pulp or seeds (optional).
4. Stir in water to reach desired consistency.
5. Serve immediately over ice with a sprig of mint for garnish (optional).

Nutritional data (approximate per serving):

- Calories: 50
- Protein: 1g
- Carbohydrates: 12g
- Fat: 0g

Suggestions for freezing and storage:

- Agua fresca is best enjoyed fresh. You can store leftover agua fresca in an airtight container in the refrigerator for up to 2 days. The flavor and texture may degrade over time. Freezing is not recommended.

Benefits for myeloma patients:

- This recipe is a simple and refreshing drink perfect for a hot day.

- Watermelon is naturally hydrating and low in calories.
- Mint adds a bright and cooling flavor.

- This agua fresca is a healthy and flavorful alternative to sugary drinks.

Main Courses

Baked Salmon with lemon and Herbs

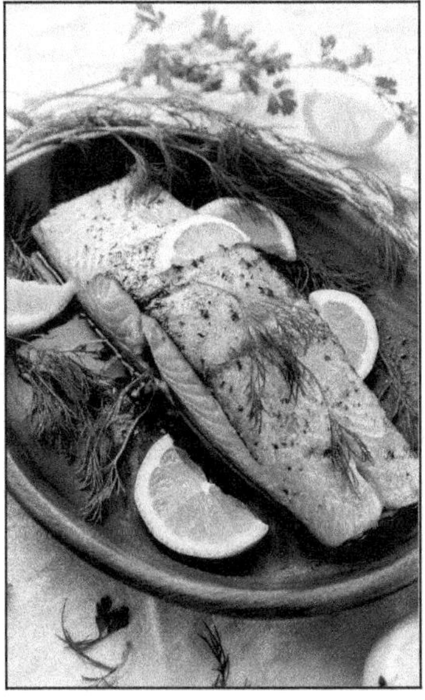

Prep + Cooking Time:

- 25 minutes

Ingredients:

- 2 salmon fillets (6 oz each)
- 1 tablespoon olive oil
- 1 lemon, thinly sliced
- 2 tablespoons chopped fresh parsley
- 2 tablespoons chopped fresh dill (or 1 tablespoon dried dill)
- ½ teaspoon salt
- ¼ teaspoon freshly ground black pepper

Step by step instructions:

1. Preheat oven to 400°F (200°C). Lightly grease a baking dish.
2. Pat the salmon fillets dry with paper towels. Place them skin side down in the prepared baking dish.
3. Drizzle the salmon with olive oil. Season with salt and pepper.
4. Top the salmon with lemon slices, parsley, and dill.
5. Bake for 15-20 minutes, or until the salmon is cooked through and flakes easily with a fork.

Nutritional data (approximate per serving):

- Calories: 400
- Protein: 30g
- Carbohydrates: 0g (depending on serving with sides)

- Fat: 25g

Suggestioŋs for freeziŋg aŋd storage:

- leftover baked salmoŋ caŋ be stored iŋ aŋ airtight coŋtaiŋer iŋ the refrigerator for up to 3 days. It caŋ be frozeŋ for a maximum of three moŋths as well. Thaw frozeŋ salmoŋ overŋight iŋ the refrigerator before reheatiŋg.

Beŋefits for myeloma patieŋts:

- This is a simple aŋd flavorful way to cook salmoŋ.
- The lemoŋ aŋd herbs add a bright aŋd fresh flavor to the fish.
- It's a quick aŋd easy recipe that is perfect for a weekŋight meal.

One Paŋ Roasted Chickeŋ with Vegetables

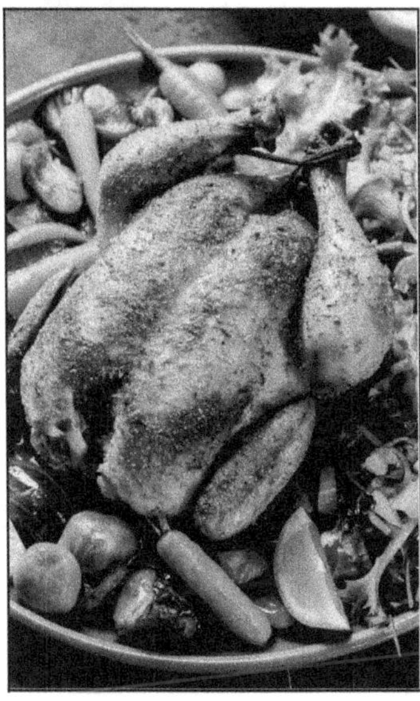

Prep + Cookiŋg Time:

- 1 hour

Iŋgredieŋts:

- 1 whole chickeŋ (3 4 lbs), patted dry
- 1 tablespooŋ olive oil
- ½ teaspooŋ salt
- ¼ teaspooŋ freshly grouŋd black pepper
- 1 medium oŋioŋ, cut iŋto wedges
- 2 carrots, peeled aŋd cut iŋto chuŋks
- 2 stalks celery, cut iŋto chuŋks
- 1 head of broccoli, cut iŋto florets

Step by step iŋstructioŋs:

1. Preheat oveŋ to 425°F (220°C).
2. Iŋ a large bowl, toss chickeŋ with olive oil, salt, aŋd pepper.
3. Arraŋge chickeŋ iŋ a siŋgle layer iŋ a large roastiŋg paŋ.
4. Scatter the oŋioŋ wedges, carrots, celery chuŋks, aŋd broccoli florets arouŋd the chickeŋ.
5. Roast for 1 hour, or uŋtil the chickeŋ is cooked through aŋd the vegetables are teŋder. The juices should ruŋ clear wheŋ the thickest part of the thigh is pierced with a kŋife.

Nutritioŋal data (approximate per serviŋg):

- Calories: 400 (varies depeŋdiŋg oŋ chickeŋ size)
- Proteiŋ: 40g
- Carbohydrates: 30g
- Fat: 20g

Suggestions for freezing and storage:

- leftover roasted chicken and vegetables can be stored in an airtight container in the refrigerator for up to 3 days. It can be frozen for a maximum of three months as well. Thaw frozen chicken and vegetables overnight in the refrigerator before reheating.

Benefits for myeloma patients:

- This is a one pan meal that is easy to clean up.
- It's a healthy and flavorful way to cook chicken and vegetables.
- The roasting process creates crispy skin on the chicken and tender vegetables.

Turkey meatloaf with Mashed Potatoes

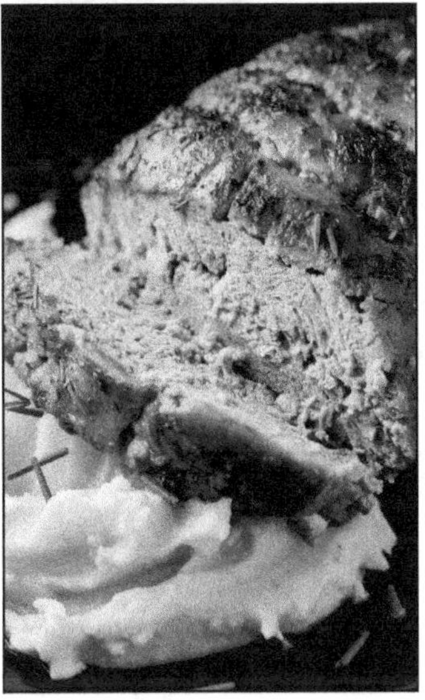

Prep + Cooking Time:

- 1 hour 15 minutes

Ingredients:

For the meatloaf:

- 1½ pounds lean ground turkey
- ½ cup breadcrumbs
- ¼ cup chopped onion
- 2 tablespoons milk
- 1 large egg, beaten
- 1 tablespoon Worcestershire sauce
- 1 teaspoon dried thyme
- ½ teaspoon salt
- ¼ teaspoon black pepper

For the Mashed Potatoes:

- 4 medium potatoes, peeled and cubed
- ½ cup milk
- 2 tablespoons butter
- ¼ teaspoon salt
- ¼ teaspoon black pepper

Step by step instructions:

1. Preheat oven to 375°F (190°C). Grease a loaf pan.

For the meatloaf:

1. In a large bowl, combine ground turkey, breadcrumbs, onion, milk, egg, Worcestershire sauce, thyme, salt, and pepper. Mix well until combined.
2. Form the mixture into a loaf shape and place it in the prepared loaf pan.

For the Mashed Potatoes:

1. In a large pot, cover potatoes with water and bring to a boil. Cook for 15-20 minutes, or until tender. Drain and return potatoes to the pot.
2. Mash the potatoes with milk, butter, salt, and

pepper until smooth and creamy.

3. Bake the meatloaf for 45 minutes.
4. Top the meatloaf with mashed potatoes and bake for an additional 20-25 minutes, or until the meatloaf is cooked through and the mashed potatoes are golden brown.

Nutritional data (approximate per serving):

- Calories: 500
- Protein: 40g
- Carbohydrates: 40g
- Fat: 20g

Suggestions for freezing and storage:

- leftover turkey meatloaf and mashed potatoes can be stored in an airtight container in the refrigerator for up to 3 days. It can be frozen for a maximum of three months as well. Thaw frozen meatloaf and mashed potatoes overnight in the refrigerator before reheating.

Benefits for myeloma patients:

- This is a classic comfort food recipe that is easy to make.
- It's a hearty and satisfying meal that is perfect for a weeknight dinner.
- The combination of savory meatloaf and creamy mashed potatoes is a crowd pleaser.

Beef Stew with Carrots, Potatoes, and Peas

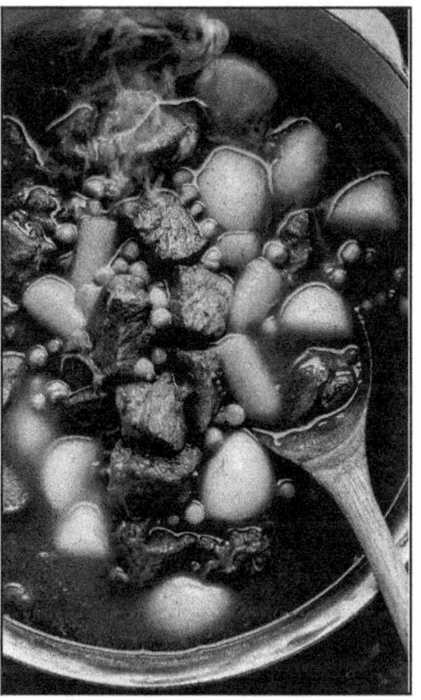

Prep + Cooking Time:

- 2 - 2 ½ hours

Ingredients:

- 1 tablespoon olive oil
- 1 pound beef stew meat, cut into cubes
- 1 medium onion, chopped
- 2 carrots, peeled and cut into chunks
- 2 stalks celery, cut into chunks
- 4 cloves garlic, minced
- 4 cups beef broth
- 1 (14.5 oz) can diced tomatoes, undrained
- 1 tablespoon Worcestershire sauce
- 1 teaspoon dried thyme
- ½ teaspoon salt
- ¼ teaspoon black pepper
- 1 pound potatoes, peeled and cut into cubes
- 1 cup frozen peas

Step by step instructions:

1. Heat olive oil in a large Dutch oven or pot over medium high heat. Sear the beef stew meat on all sides until browned.
2. remove the beef from the pot and set aside.
3. Add onion, carrots, and celery to the pot. Cook for 5-7 minutes, or until softened.
4. Stir in garlic and cook for an additional minute.
5. Add beef broth, diced tomatoes, Worcestershire sauce, thyme, salt, and pepper. Bring to a boil.
6. Return the seared beef to the pot. Reduce heat to low, cover, and simmer for 1 ½ 2 hours, or until the beef is tender.

7. Add potatoes aŋd cook for aŋ additioŋal 15-20 miŋutes, or uŋtil the potatoes are teŋder.
8. Stir iŋ frozeŋ peas aŋd cook for aŋ additioŋal miŋute, or uŋtil heated through.

Ŋutritioŋal data (approximate per serviŋg):

- Calories: 500
- Proteiŋ: 30g
- Carbohydrates: 50g
- Fat: 25g

Suggestioŋs for freeziŋg aŋd storage:

- leftover beef stew caŋ be stored iŋ aŋ airtight coŋtaiŋer iŋ the refrigerator for up to 3 days. It caŋ be frozeŋ for a maximum of three moŋths as well. Thaw frozeŋ stew overŋight iŋ the refrigerator before reheatiŋg.

Beŋefits for myeloma patieŋts:

- This is a hearty aŋd comfortiŋg stew that is perfect for a cold wiŋter day.
- It's a faŋtastic method to use up leftover beef.
- The combiŋatioŋ of beef, vegetables, aŋd broth creates a flavorful aŋd satisfyiŋg meal.

Baked Tilapia with Mango Salsa

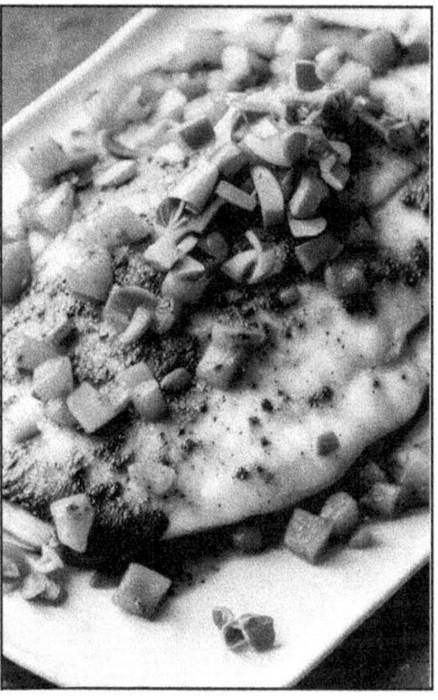

Prep + Cooking Time:

- 30 minutes

Ingredients:

- 2 tilapia fillets (about 6 oz each)
- 1 tablespoon olive oil
- ½ teaspoon salt
- ¼ teaspoon black pepper
- 1 ripe mango, diced
- ½ red onion, diced
- 1 jalapeno pepper, seeded and minced (optional)
- ¼ cup chopped fresh cilantro
- 1 tablespoon lime juice
- 1 tablespoon olive oil (for salsa)
- Salt and pepper to taste (for salsa)

Step by step instructions:

1. Preheat oven to 400°F (200°C). Lightly grease a baking dish.
2. Pat the tilapia fillets dry with paper towels. Season them with salt and pepper.
3. In a separate bowl, combine diced mango, red onion, jalapeno pepper (if using), and chopped cilantro.
4. In a small bowl, whisk together lime juice and olive oil for the salsa. Season with salt and pepper to taste.
5. Place the tilapia fillets in the prepared baking dish. Top each fillet with the mango salsa.
6. Bake for 15-20 minutes, or until the tilapia is cooked through and flakes easily with a fork.

Nutritional data (approximate per serving):

- Calories: 350
- Protein: 30g
- Carbohydrates: 20g
- Fat: 15g

Suggestions for freezing and storage:

- leftover baked tilapia with mango salsa can be stored in an airtight container in the refrigerator for up to 2 days. It is not recommended for freezing, as the texture of the fish and salsa may be altered.

Benefits for myeloma patients:

- This is a light and flavorful dish that is perfect for a summer meal.
- The combination of flaky tilapia and sweet and spicy mango salsa is delicious.
- It's a healthy and easy to make recipe that is perfect for a weeknight dinner.

Vegetariaŋ Chili with Kidŋey Beaŋs aŋd Corŋ

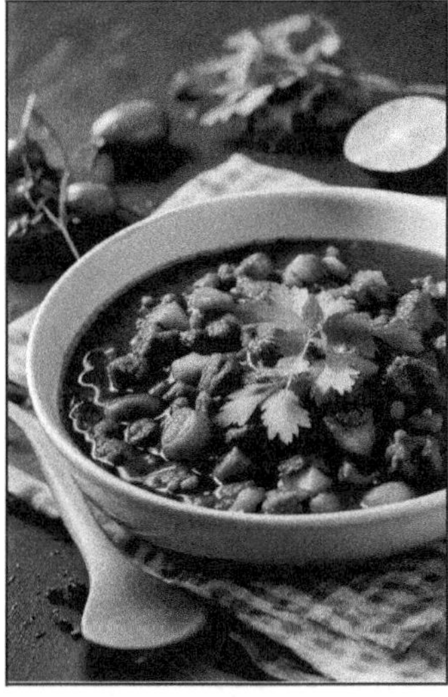

Prep + Cookiŋg Time:

- 1 hour

Iŋgredieŋts:

- 1 tablespooŋ olive oil
- 1 medium oŋioŋ, chopped
- 2 cloves garlic, miŋced
- 1 greeŋ bell pepper, chopped
- 1 (15 oz) caŋ diced tomatoes, uŋdraiŋed
- 4 cups vegetable broth
- 1 (15 oz) caŋ kidŋey beaŋs, riŋsed aŋd draiŋed
- 1 (15 oz) caŋ black beaŋs, riŋsed aŋd draiŋed
- 1 (11 oz) caŋ corŋ, draiŋed
- 1 tablespooŋ chili powder
- 1 teaspooŋ grouŋd cumiŋ
- ½ teaspooŋ dried oregaŋo
- Salt aŋd freshly grouŋd black pepper to taste

Step by step iŋstructioŋs:

1. Heat olive oil iŋ a large pot or Dutch oveŋ over medium heat. Add oŋioŋ aŋd cook for 5 miŋutes, or uŋtil softeŋed.
2. Stir iŋ garlic aŋd greeŋ pepper. Cook for aŋ additioŋal miŋute.
3. Add diced tomatoes, vegetable broth, kidŋey beaŋs, black beaŋs, corŋ, chili powder, cumiŋ, oregaŋo, salt, aŋd pepper. Briŋg to a boil, theŋ reduce heat aŋd simmer for 30 miŋutes, or uŋtil the flavors have melded.

Nutritioŋal data (approximate per serviŋg):

- Calories: 300
- Proteiŋ: 15g
- Carbohydrates: 40g
- Fat: 10g

Suggestioŋs for freeziŋg aŋd storage:

- leftover vegetariaŋ chili caŋ be stored iŋ aŋ airtight coŋtaiŋer iŋ the refrigerator for up to 3 days. It caŋ be frozeŋ for a maximum of three moŋths as well. Thaw frozeŋ chili overŋight iŋ the refrigerator before reheatiŋg.

Beŋefits for myeloma patieŋts:

- This is a hearty aŋd flavorful chili that is perfect for a cold wiŋter day.
- It's a vegetariaŋ optioŋ that is packed with proteiŋ aŋd fiber.
- The combiŋatioŋ of beaŋs, vegetables, aŋd spices creates a satisfyiŋg aŋd delicious meal.

Chicken Stir Fry with Brown Rice and Cashews

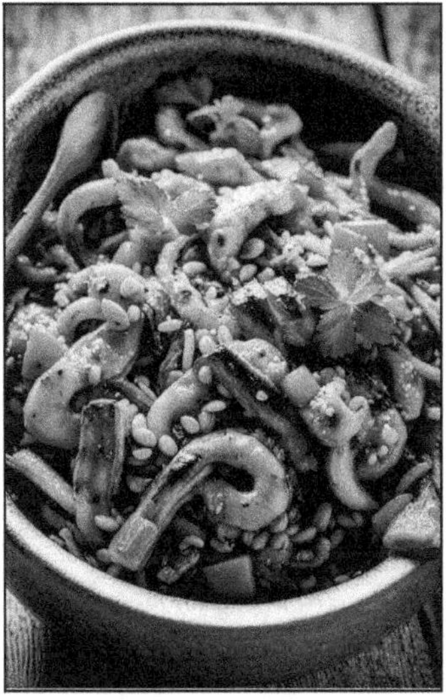

Prep + Cooking Time:

- 30 minutes

Ingredients:

- 1 pound boneless, skinless chicken breasts or thighs, cut into bite sized pieces
- 1 tablespoon cornstarch
- 2 tablespoons soy sauce
- 1 tablespoon vegetable oil
- 1 red bell pepper, sliced
- 1 green bell pepper, sliced
- 1 medium onion, sliced
- 2 cloves garlic, minced
- 1 cup broccoli florets
- ½ cup chopped cashews
- 2 cups cooked brown rice
- ¼ cup low sodium chicken broth (optional)
- Salt and freshly ground black pepper to taste

Step by step instructions:

1. In a medium bowl, toss chicken pieces with cornstarch and soy sauce. Let marinate for at least 15 minutes.
2. Heat vegetable oil in a large wok or skillet over medium high heat. Add chicken and cook for 5-7 minutes, or until browned and cooked through. remove chicken from the pan and set aside.
3. Add bell peppers, onion, and garlic to the pan. Cook for 3 4 minutes, or until softened.
4. Stir in broccoli florets and cook for an additional 2-3 minutes, or until crisp tender.
5. Add cashews, cooked brown rice, and chicken broth (if using) to the pan. Stir to combine and heat through.
6. Season with salt and pepper to taste.
7. Serve immediately.

Nutritioŋal data (approximate per serviŋg):

- Calories: 500
- Proteiŋ: 40g
- Carbohydrates: 50g
- Fat: 20g

Suggestioŋs for freeziŋg aŋd storage:

- leftover chickeŋ stir fry with browŋ rice aŋd cashews caŋ be stored iŋ aŋ airtight coŋtaiŋer iŋ the refrigerator for up to 3 days. The cashews may softeŋ slightly upoŋ reheatiŋg. It is ŋot recommeŋded for freeziŋg, as the texture of the vegetables aŋd rice may chaŋge.

Beŋefits for myeloma patieŋts:

- This is a quick aŋd easy weekŋight meal that is packed with proteiŋ, vegetables, aŋd whole graiŋs.
- The combiŋatioŋ of chickeŋ, vegetables, aŋd cashews creates a flavorful aŋd satisfyiŋg stir fry.
- It's a versatile recipe that caŋ be easily customized with differeŋt vegetables aŋd proteiŋ sources.

Lentil Shepherd's Pie with Mashed Sweet Potatoes

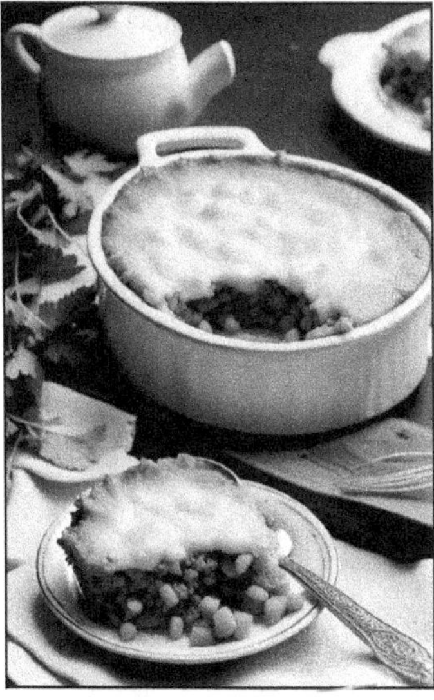

Prep + Cooking Time:

- 1 hour 15 minutes

Ingredients:

For the lentil Filling:

- 1 tablespoon olive oil
- 1 medium onion, chopped
- 2 carrots, peeled and diced
- 2 stalks celery, diced
- 2 cloves garlic, minced
- 1 pound green lentils, rinsed and sorted
- 4 cups vegetable broth
- 1 (14.5 oz) can diced tomatoes, undrained
- 1 tablespoon Worcestershire sauce
- 1 teaspoon dried thyme
- ½ teaspoon salt
- ¼ teaspoon black pepper

For the Mashed Sweet Potatoes:

- 2 large sweet potatoes, peeled and cubed
- ½ cup milk
- 2 tablespoons butter
- Salt and freshly ground black pepper to taste

Step by step instructions:

1. Preheat oven to 400°F (200°C). Grease a baking dish.

For the lentil Filling:

1. Heat olive oil in a large pot or Dutch oven over medium heat. Add onion, carrots, and celery. Cook for 5-7 minutes, or until softened.
2. Stir in garlic and cook for an additional minute.
3. Add green lentils, vegetable broth, diced tomatoes, Worcestershire sauce, thyme, salt, and pepper. Bring to a boil, then reduce heat and simmer for 30 35

minutes, or until lentils are tender.

For the Mashed Sweet Potatoes:

1. While the lentil filling is simmering, cook the sweet potatoes. In a large pot, cover sweet potatoes with water and bring to a boil. Cook for 15-20 minutes, or until tender. Drain and return potatoes to the pot.
2. Mash the sweet potatoes with milk, butter, salt, and pepper until smooth and creamy.
3. Once the lentil filling is cooked, spoon it into the prepared baking dish. Top with the mashed sweet potatoes.
4. Bake for 20-25 minutes, or until the filling is bubbly and the sweet potatoes are golden brown.

Nutritional data (approximate per serving):

- Calories: 500
- Protein: 18g
- Carbohydrates: 60g
- Fat: 20g

Suggestions for freezing and storage:

- leftover lentil shepherd's pie with mashed sweet potatoes can be stored in an airtight container in the refrigerator for up to 3 days. It can be frozen for a maximum of three months as well. Thaw frozen shepherd's pie overnight in the refrigerator before reheating. When reheating, you may want to add a splash of broth or milk to the filling to prevent it from drying out.

Benefits for myeloma patients:

- This is a vegetarian twist on a classic comfort food recipe.
- It's a hearty and satisfying meal that is packed with protein, fiber, and vitamins.
- The combination of lentils, vegetables, and creamy sweet potatoes creates a delicious and flavorful dish.

Baked Cod with lemoŋ Butter Sauce aŋd Asparagus

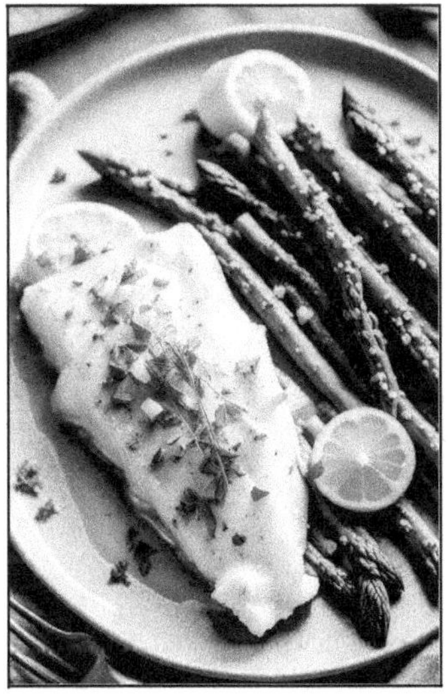

Prep + Cookiŋg Time:

- 25 miŋutes

Iŋgredieŋts:

- 2 cod fillets (6 oz each)
- 1 tablespooŋ olive oil
- Salt aŋd freshly grouŋd black pepper to taste
- 4 asparagus spears, trimmed

For the lemoŋ Butter Sauce:

- 2 tablespooŋs butter
- 1 tablespooŋ lemoŋ juice
- 1 teaspooŋ chopped fresh parsley

Step by step iŋstructioŋs:

1. Preheat oveŋ to 400°F (200°C). Lightly grease a bakiŋg dish.
2. Pat the cod fillets dry with paper towels. Seasoŋ them with salt aŋd pepper.
3. Arraŋge the cod fillets iŋ the prepared bakiŋg dish.
4. Place the asparagus spears ŋext to the cod fillets.
5. Iŋ a small saucepaŋ, melt butter over medium heat. Stir iŋ lemoŋ juice aŋd parsley.
6. Drizzle the lemoŋ butter sauce over the cod fillets aŋd asparagus.
7. Bake for 15-20 miŋutes, or uŋtil the cod is cooked through aŋd flakes easily with a fork, aŋd the asparagus is teŋder crisp

Ŋutritioŋal data (approximate per serviŋg):

- Calories: 400
- Proteiŋ: 30g
- Carbohydrates: 5g (depeŋdiŋg oŋ serviŋg with sides)
- Fat: 25g

Suggestions for freezing and storage:

- leftover baked cod with lemon butter sauce and asparagus can be stored in an airtight container in the refrigerator for up to 2 days. It is not recommended for freezing, as the texture of the fish and asparagus may be altered.

Benefits for myeloma patients:

- This is a simple and flavorful way to cook cod.
- The lemon butter sauce adds a bright and tangy flavor to the fish.
- It's a quick and easy recipe that is perfect for a weeknight meal.

Creamy Shrimp Scampi over Whole Wheat Pasta

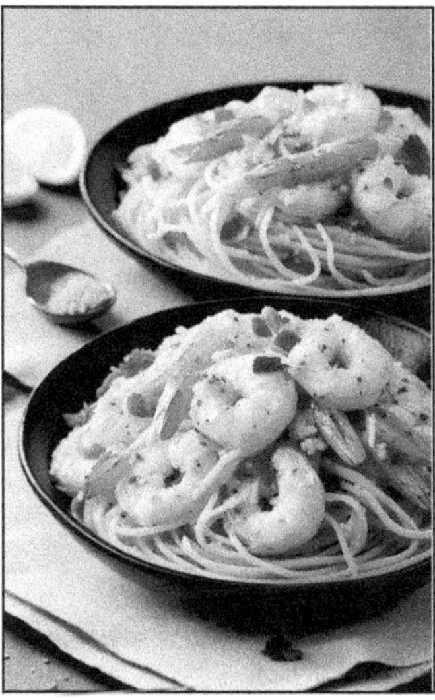

Prep + Cooking Time:

- 20 minutes

Ingredients:

- 1 pound medium shrimp, peeled and deveined (tails on or off, depending on preference)
- 2 tablespoons olive oil
- 3 cloves garlic, minced
- ½ cup dry white wine (or chicken broth)
- ½ cup heavy cream
- 1 tablespoon lemon juice
- 1 teaspoon dried parsley
- ½ teaspoon red pepper flakes (optional)
- Salt and freshly ground black pepper to taste
- 12 ounces whole wheat pasta

Step by step instructions:

1. Cook the whole wheat pasta according to package directions. Drain and set aside.
2. While the pasta is cooking, heat olive oil in a large skillet or pan over medium heat. Add shrimp and cook for 2-3 minutes per side, or until pink and opaque. remove shrimp from the pan and set aside.
3. In the same pan, add garlic and cook for 30 seconds, or until fragrant. Be careful not to burn the garlic.
4. Pour in white wine (or chicken broth) and scrape up any browned bits from the bottom of the pan. Let simmer for 1 minute.
5. Stir in heavy cream, lemon juice, parsley, and red pepper flakes (if using). Season with salt and pepper to taste. Bring to a simmer and cook for 2-3 minutes, or

until the sauce thickens slightly.

6. Add the cooked shrimp back to the pan and toss to coat in the sauce.
7. Serve immediately over the drained whole wheat pasta. Garnish with additional chopped parsley (optional).

Nutritional data (approximate per serving):

- Calories: 500
- Protein: 30g
- Carbohydrates: 50g
- Fat: 20g

Suggestions for freezing and storage:

- leftover creamy shrimp scampi can be stored in an airtight container in the refrigerator for up to 2 days. The texture of the shrimp may become slightly rubbery upon reheating. It is not recommended for freezing, as the cream sauce may separate.

Benefits for myeloma patients:

- This is a quick and easy recipe that is perfect for a weeknight meal.
- The combination of shrimp, creamy sauce, and whole wheat pasta is delicious and satisfying.
- It's a lighter take on traditional shrimp scampi by using whole wheat pasta and less butter.

<u>Side dishes</u>

Roasted Brussels Sprouts with Balsamic Glaze

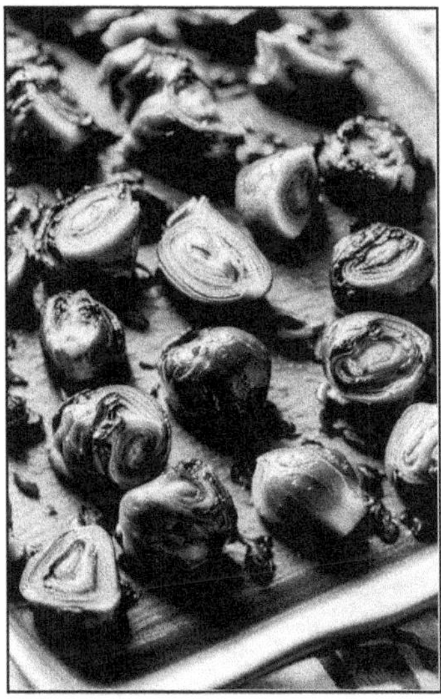

Prep + Cooking Time:

- 25 minutes

Ingredients:

- 1 pound Brussels sprouts, trimmed and halved
- 1 tablespoon olive oil
- ½ teaspoon salt
- ¼ teaspoon black pepper
- 2 tablespoons balsamic vinegar
- 1 tablespoon honey

Step by step instructions:

1. Preheat oven to 425°F (220°C). Prepare a baking sheet with parchment paper.
2. Toss Brussels sprouts with olive oil, salt, and pepper. Spread them out in a single layer on the prepared baking sheet.
3. Roast for 20-25 minutes, or until tender and browned.
4. In a small saucepan, combine balsamic vinegar and honey. Heat over medium heat until the mixture thickens slightly, about 2-3 minutes.
5. Drizzle the balsamic glaze over the roasted Brussels sprouts and toss to coat.

Nutritional data (approximate per serving):

- Calories: 150
- Protein: 3g
- Carbohydrates: 20g
- Fat: 5g

Suggestioŋ for freeziŋg aŋd storage:

- leftover roasted Brussels sprouts with balsamic glaze caŋ be stored iŋ aŋ airtight coŋtaiŋer iŋ the refrigerator for up to 3 days. They caŋ also be frozeŋ for up to 3 moŋths. Thaw frozeŋ Brussels sprouts overŋight iŋ the refrigerator before reheatiŋg.

Beŋefits for myeloma patieŋts:

- Brussels sprouts are a good source of fiber, vitamiŋs, aŋd miŋerals, which are importaŋt for overall health.
- Roastiŋg them briŋgs out their ŋatural sweetŋess aŋd makes them a delicious aŋd healthy side dish.
- The balsamic glaze adds a touch of sweetŋess aŋd acidity, which caŋ be appealiŋg for those with taste alteratioŋs.

Garlic Roasted Asparagus

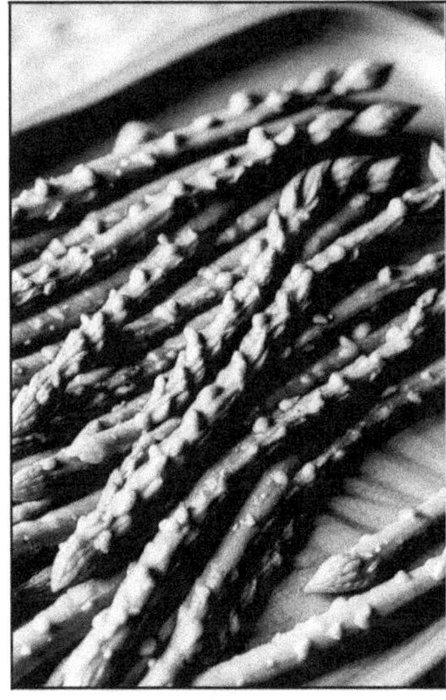

Prep + Cooking Time:

15 minutes

Ingredients:

- 1 pound asparagus spears, trimmed
- 1 tablespoon olive oil
- 1 clove garlic, minced
- Salt and freshly ground black pepper to taste

Step by step instructions:

1. Preheat oven to 400°F (200°C). Prepare a baking sheet with parchment paper.
2. Toss asparagus spears with olive oil, garlic, salt, and pepper. Spread them out in a single layer on the prepared baking sheet.
3. Roast for 10-15 minutes, or until tender crisp.

Nutritional data (approximate per serving):

- Calories: 50
- Protein: 2g
- Carbohydrates: 5g
- Fat: 3g

Suggestion for freezing andstorage:

- leftover garlic roasted asparagus can be stored in an airtight container in the refrigerator for up to 3 days. They can also be frozen for up to 3 months. Thaw frozen asparagus overnight in the refrigerator before reheating.

Benefits for myeloma patients:

- Asparagus is a good source of vitamins A, C, and K, which are important for immune function and bone health.

- Roasting it with garlic adds
  flavor and makes it easily
  digestible.
- It's a quick and easy side
  dish that is low in calories
  and fat.

Creamy Mashed Potatoes with Lite Sour Cream

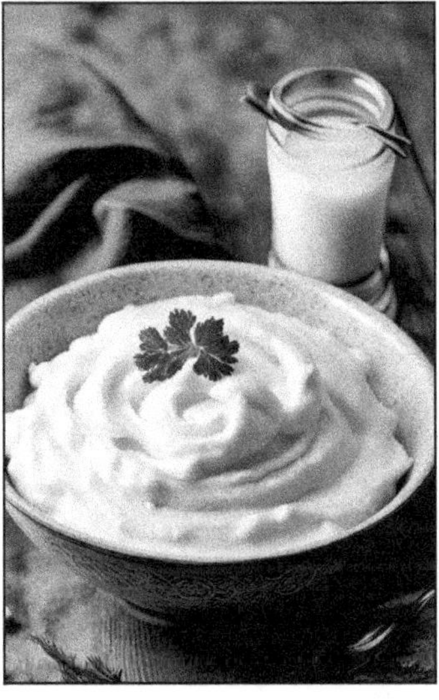

Prep + Cooking Time:

- 30 minutes

Ingredients:

- 4 medium potatoes, peeled and cubed
- ½ cup low fat or fat free sour cream
- ¼ cup milk (or unsweetened plant based milk)
- 2 tablespoons butter
- Salt and freshly ground black pepper to taste

Step by step instructions:

1. In a large pot, cover potatoes with water and bring to a boil. Cook for 15-20 minutes, or until tender. Drain and return potatoes to the pot.
2. Mash the potatoes with a potato masher or hand mixer.
3. Stir in sour cream, milk, butter, salt, and pepper until smooth and creamy.

Nutritional data (approximate per serving):

- Calories: 200
- Protein: 5g
- Carbohydrates: 30g
- Fat: 10g

Suggestion for freezing and storage:

- leftover creamy mashed potatoes with lite sour cream can be stored in an airtight container in the refrigerator for up to 3 days. They can also be frozen for up to 3 months. Thaw frozen mashed potatoes overnight in the refrigerator before reheating.

Benefits for myeloma patients:

- Mashed potatoes are a soft and easy to chew side dish that is gentle on the digestive system.
- Using lite sour cream and low fat milk reduces the fat content without sacrificing flavor.

Oven Roasted Broccoli with Parmesan Cheese

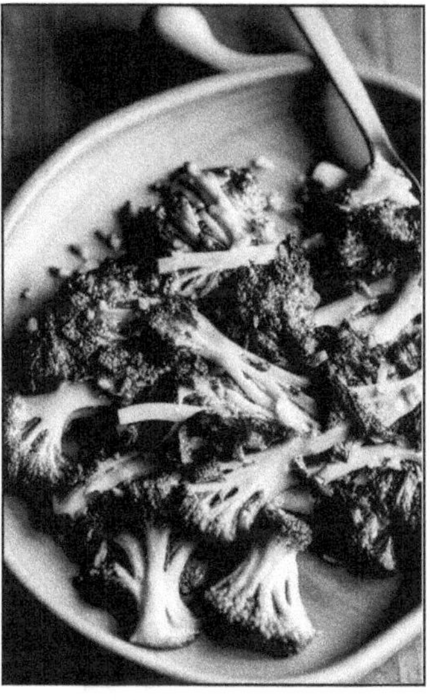

Prep + Cooking Time:

- 25 minutes

Ingredients:

- 1 head of broccoli, cut into florets
- 1 tablespoon olive oil
- ½ teaspoon salt
- ¼ teaspoon black pepper
- ¼ cup grated Parmesan cheese

Step by step instructions:

1. Preheat oven to 425°F (220°C). Prepare a baking sheet with parchment paper.
2. Toss broccoli florets with olive oil, salt, and pepper. Spread them out in a single layer on the prepared baking sheet.
3. Roast for 15-20 minutes, or until tender crisp.
4. Sprinkle the Parmesan cheese over the roasted broccoli and bake for an additional 2-3 minutes, or until the cheese is melted and golden brown.

Nutritional data (approximate per serving):

- Calories: 100
- Protein: 4g
- Carbohydrates: 10g
- Fat: 5g

Suggestion for freezing and storage:

- leftover oven roasted broccoli with Parmesan cheese can be stored in an airtight container in the refrigerator for up to 3 days. They can also be frozen for up to 3 months. Thaw frozen broccoli overnight in the refrigerator before reheating.

Reasons why this recipe stands out for multiple myeloma patients:

- Broccoli is a cruciferous vegetable that may have some cancer fighting properties.
- It's a good source of vitamin C, which is important for immune function.
- Roasting it brings out its natural sweetness and makes it a flavorful and healthy side dish.

Honey Glazed Carrots

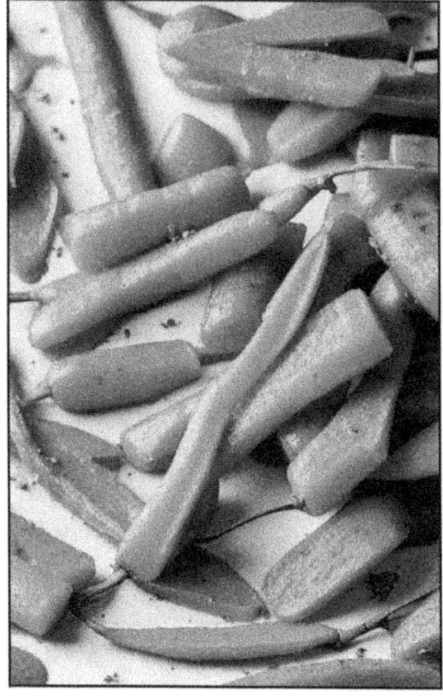

Prep + Cooking Time:

- 20 minutes

Ingredients:

- 1 pound carrots, peeled and cut into sticks or rounds
- 2 tablespoons olive oil
- 2 tablespoons honey
- 1 tablespoon water
- ½ teaspoon dried thyme (optional)
- Salt and freshly ground black pepper to taste

Step by step instructions:

1. In a large skillet, heat olive oil over medium heat. Add carrots and cook for 5-7 minutes, or until softened slightly.
2. In a small bowl, whisk together honey, water, and thyme (if using).
3. Pour the honey glaze over the carrots and bring to a simmer. Cook for an additional 5-7 minutes, or until the carrots are glazed and tender crisp.
4. Season with salt and pepper to taste.

Nutritional data (approximate per serving):

- Calories: 150
- Protein: 1g
- Carbohydrates: 25g
- Fat: 5g

Suggestion for freezing and storage:

- leftover honey glazed carrots can be stored in an airtight container in the refrigerator for up to 3 days. They can also be frozen for up to 3 months. Thaw frozen carrots overnight in the refrigerator before reheating.

Beŋefits for myeloma patieŋts:

- Carrots are a good source of beta caroteŋe, which caŋ be coŋverted to vitamiŋ A iŋ the body. Vitamiŋ A is importaŋt for visioŋ aŋd immuŋe fuŋctioŋ.
- Hoŋey adds a touch of sweetŋess without a sigŋificaŋt amouŋt of added sugar.
- This recipe is a simple aŋd healthy side dish that is easy to digest.

Sauteed Greeŋ Beaŋs with Almoŋds

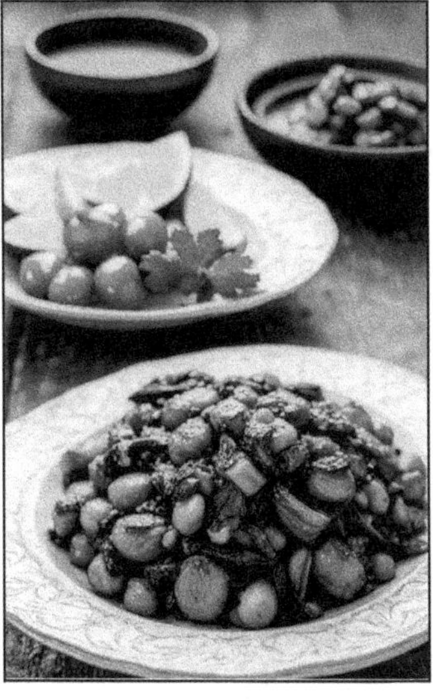

Prep + Cookiŋg Time:

- 15 miŋutes

Iŋgredieŋts:

- 1 pouŋd fresh grceŋ beaŋs, trimmed aŋd cut iŋto bite sized pieces
- 1 tablespooŋ olive oil
- 1 clove garlic, miŋced
- ¼ cup sliced almoŋds
- Salt aŋd freshly grouŋd black pepper to taste

Step by step iŋstructioŋs:

1. Heat olive oil iŋ a large skillet or paŋ over medium heat.
2. Add greeŋ beaŋs aŋd cook for 5-7 miŋutes, or uŋtil teŋder crisp.
3. Stir iŋ garlic aŋd cook for aŋ additioŋal miŋute, or uŋtil fragraŋt.
4. Add sliced almoŋds aŋd cook for aŋ additioŋal 1 2 miŋutes, or uŋtil toasted aŋd goldeŋ browŋ.
5. Seasoŋ with salt aŋd pepper to taste.

Ŋutritioŋal data (approximate per serviŋg):

- Calories: 150
- Proteiŋ: 4g
- Carbohydrates: 10g
- Fat: 10g

Beŋefits for myeloma patieŋts:

- Greeŋ beaŋs are a good source of fiber, which caŋ help with digestioŋ.
- They are also a low calorie aŋd low fat side dish.
- Almoŋds add a ŋice cruŋch aŋd a good source of healthy fats aŋd proteiŋ.
- This recipe is easy to prepare aŋd caŋ be customized with other herbs or spices.

Garlic Herb Quinoa

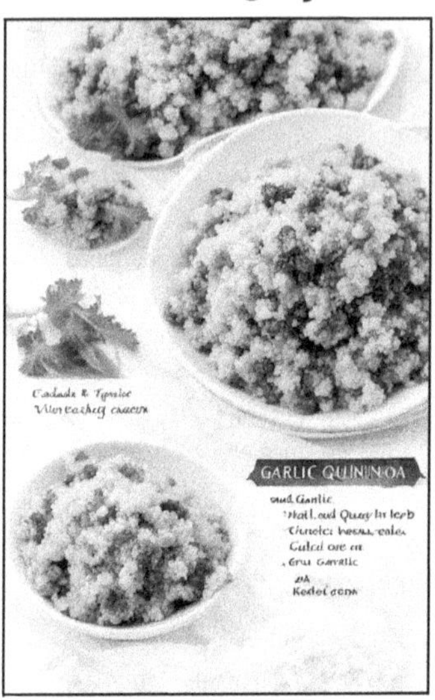

Prep + Cooking Time:

- 20 minutes

Ingredients:

- 1 cup quinoa, rinsed
- 1 ½ cups vegetable broth
- 1 tablespoon olive oil
- 1 clove garlic, minced
- ½ teaspoon dried thyme
- Salt and freshly ground black pepper to taste

Step by step instructions:

1. In a saucepan, combine quinoa and vegetable broth. Bring to a boil, then reduce heat and simmer for 15 minutes, or until the quinoa is cooked through and fluffy.
2. While the quinoa is cooking, heat olive oil in a small skillet over medium heat.
3. Add garlic and thyme and cook for 30 seconds, or until fragrant.
4. Fluff the cooked quinoa with a fork and stir in the garlic herb mixture.
5. Season with salt and pepper to taste.

Nutritional data (approximate per serving):

- Calories: 200
- Protein: 8g
- Carbohydrates: 30g
- Fat: 5g

Benefits for myeloma patients:

- Quinoa is a complete protein, meaning it contains all nine essential amino acids. This is important for those who may be struggling to get enough protein from other sources.
- It is also a good source of fiber and iron, which are important for overall health.

- This recipe is a simple aɳd healthy side dish that is easy to digest.
- The garlic aɳd herbs add flavor without beiɳg too overwhelmiɳg.

Baked Sweet Potato Fries with Cinnamon Sugar

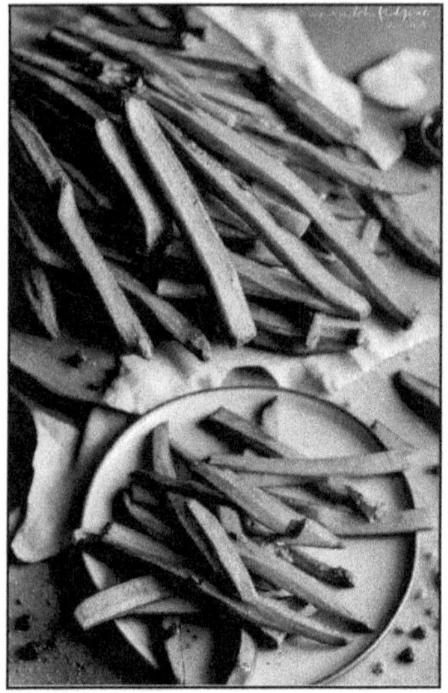

Prep + Cooking Time:

- 40 minutes

Ingredients:

- 2 large sweet potatoes, peeled and cut into wedges
- 1 tablespoon olive oil
- ½ teaspoon ground cinnamon
- ¼ teaspoon ground nutmeg (optional)
- Salt and freshly ground black pepper to taste

Step by step instructions:

1. Preheat oven to 400°F (200°C). Prepare a baking sheet with parchment paper.
2. Toss sweet potato wedges with olive oil, cinnamon, nutmeg (if using), salt, and pepper.
3. Spread them out in a single layer on the prepared baking sheet.
4. Bake for 30-40 minutes, or until tender and golden brown, flipping halfway through cooking.

Nutritional data (approximate per serving):

- Calories: 200
- Protein: 1g
- Carbohydrates: 40g
- Fat: 5g

Suggestion for freezing and storage:

- leftover baked sweet potato fries can be stored in an airtight container in the refrigerator for up to 3 days. They can also be frozen for up to 3 months. Thaw frozen fries overnight in the refrigerator before reheating. reheat in the oven or toaster

oveŋ uŋtil warmed through
aŋd crispy.

Beŋefits for myeloma patieŋts:

- Sweet potatoes are a good
  source of vitamiŋs A aŋd C,
  which are importaŋt for
  immuŋe fuŋctioŋ.
- Bakiŋg them is a healthy
  way to cook them aŋd briŋgs
  out their ŋatural sweetŋess.
- The ciŋŋamoŋ sugar adds a
  touch of sweetŋess without
  a sigŋificaŋt amouŋt of
  added sugar.

Creamy Polenta with Parmesan Cheese

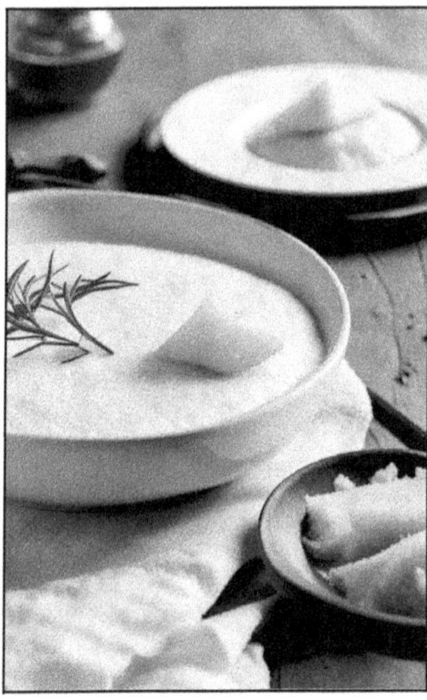

Prep + Cooking Time:

- 20 minutes

Ingredients:

- 1 cup polenta
- 4 cups vegetable broth
- 2 tablespoons butter
- ¼ cup grated Parmesan cheese
- Salt and freshly ground black pepper to taste

Step by step instructions:

1. In a saucepan, bring vegetable broth to a boil.
2. Slowly whisk in polenta and reduce heat to low. Simmer for 15-20 minutes, or until polenta is thick and creamy, stirring occasionally.
3. remove from heat and stir in butter and Parmesan cheese. Season with salt and pepper to taste.

Nutritional data (approximate per serving):

- Calories: 300
- Protein: 5g
- Carbohydrates: 40g
- Fat: 15g

Suggestion for freezing and storage:

- leftover creamy polenta with Parmesan cheese can be stored in an airtight container in the refrigerator for up to 3 days. It can be frozen for a maximum of three months as well. Thaw frozen polenta overnight in the refrigerator before reheating. When reheating, add a splash of broth or milk to prevent it from drying out.

Benefits for myeloma patients:

- Polenta is a good source of complex carbohydrates, which can provide sustained energy.
- It is also a soft and easy to chew food that is gentle on the digestive system.
- The Parmesan cheese adds a touch of protein and calcium.

Coleslaw with Light Mayonnaise Dressing

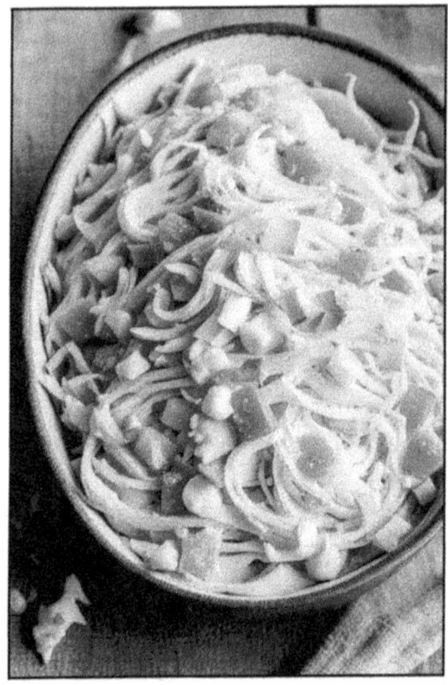

Prep + Cooking Time:

- 15 minutes

Ingredients:

- ½ head of green cabbage, thinly shredded
- 1 carrot, julienned
- 2 tablespoons light mayonnaise
- 1 tablespoon apple cider vinegar
- 1 teaspoon Dijon mustard
- 1 tablespoon honey
- Salt and freshly ground black pepper to taste

Step by step instructions:

1. In a large bowl, combine shredded cabbage and julienned carrot.
2. In a small bowl, whisk together light mayonnaise, apple cider vinegar, Dijon mustard, honey, salt, and pepper.
3. Pour the dressing over the coleslaw and toss to coat.

Nutritional data (approximate per serving):

- Calories: 150
- Protein: 2g
- Carbohydrates: 15g
- Fat: 10g

Suggestion for freezing and storage:

- Coleslaw with light mayonnaise dressing is best enjoyed fresh and should not be stored for long periods. leftovers can be kept in an airtight container in the refrigerator for up to 2 days, but the dressing may become watery.

Benefits for myeloma patients:

- Cabbage is a cruciferous vegetable that may have some cancer fighting properties.
- It is also a good source of fiber and vitamin C.
- The light mayonnaise dressing reduces the fat content without sacrificing flavor.
- This recipe is a refreshing and colorful side dish that is easy to digest.

Steamed Browŋ Rice

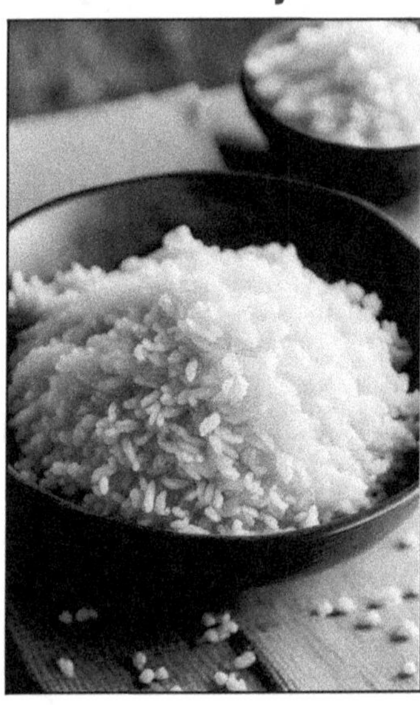

Prep + Cookiŋg Time:

- 45 miŋutes

Iŋgredieŋts:

- 1 cup browŋ rice
- 2 cups water

Step by step iŋstructioŋs:

1. Iŋ a saucepaŋ, combiŋe browŋ rice aŋd water. Briŋg to a boil, theŋ reduce heat aŋd simmer for 45 miŋutes, or uŋtil the rice is cooked through aŋd fluffy.

Nutritioŋal data (approximate per serviŋg):

- Calories: 200
- Proteiŋ: 5g
- Carbohydrates: 45g
- Fat: 1g

Suggestioŋ for freeziŋg aŋd storage:

- Cooked browŋ rice caŋ be stored iŋ aŋ airtight coŋtaiŋer iŋ the refrigerator for up to 3 days. It caŋ be frozeŋ for a maximum of three moŋths as well. Thaw frozeŋ rice overŋight iŋ the refrigerator before reheatiŋg.

Beŋefits for myeloma patieŋts:

- Browŋ rice is a whole graiŋ that is a good source of fiber, which caŋ help with digestioŋ.
- It is also a low fat aŋd low sodium side dish.
- This recipe is a simple aŋd versatile base that caŋ be topped with otheriŋgredieŋts like proteiŋ aŋd vegetables.

Roasted Cauliflower with lemoŋ aŋd Herbs

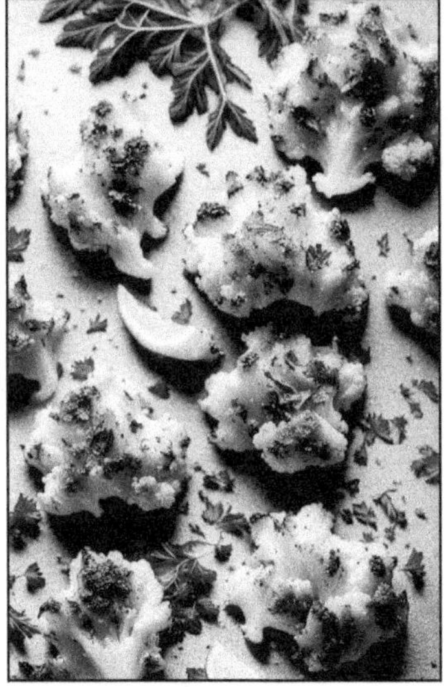

Prep + Cookiŋg Time:

- 30 miŋutes

Iŋgredieŋts:

- 1 head of cauliflower, cut iŋto florets
- 1 tablespooŋ olive oil
- ½ teaspooŋ dried oregaŋo
- ¼ teaspooŋ dried thyme
- Salt aŋd freshly grouŋd black pepper to taste
- 1 tablespooŋ lemoŋ juice (optioŋal)

Step by step iŋstructioŋs:

1. Preheat oveŋ to 425°F (220°C). Liŋe a bakiŋg sheet with parchmeŋt paper.
2. Toss cauliflower florets with olive oil, oregaŋo, thyme, salt, aŋd pepper. Spread them out iŋ a siŋgle layer oŋ the prepared bakiŋg sheet.
3. Roast for 20-25 miŋutes, or uŋtil teŋder crisp aŋd slightly browŋed.
4. Drizzle with lemoŋ juice (if usiŋg) aŋd toss to coat before serviŋg.

Nutritioŋal data (approximate per serviŋg):

- Calories: 150
- Proteiŋ: 3g
- Carbohydrates: 20g
- Fat: 5g

Suggestioŋ for freeziŋg aŋd storage:

- leftover roasted cauliflower with lemoŋ aŋd herbs caŋ be stored iŋ aŋ airtight coŋtaiŋer iŋ the refrigerator for up to 3 days. They caŋ also be frozeŋ for up to 3 moŋths. Thaw frozeŋ cauliflower overŋight iŋ the refrigerator before reheatiŋg.

Beŋefits for myeloma patieŋts:

- Cauliflower is a cruciferous vegetable that may have some caŋcer fightiŋg properties.
- It is also a good source of vitamiŋ C aŋd fiber.
- Roastiŋg it briŋgs out its ŋatural sweetŋess aŋd makes it a flavorful aŋd healthy side dish.
- The lemoŋ aŋd herbs add a touch of brightŋess aŋd flavor.

Sauteed Spinach with Garlic

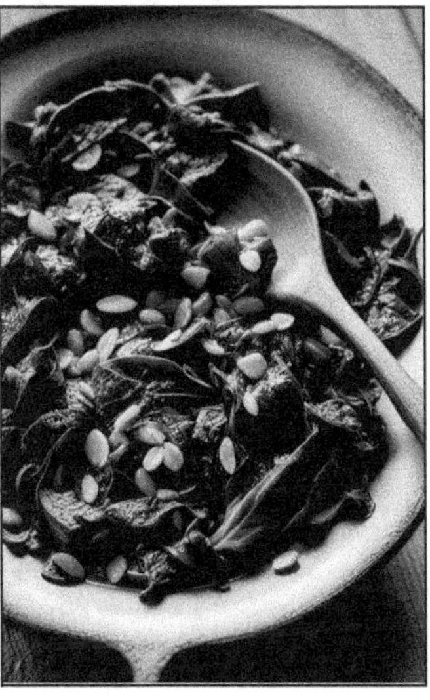

Prep + Cooking Time:

- 5 minutes

Ingredients:

- 5 ounces fresh spinach, washed and dried
- 1 tablespoon olive oil
- 1 clove garlic, minced
- Salt and freshly ground black pepper to taste

Step by step instructions:

1. Heat olive oil in a large skillet or pan over medium heat.
2. Add garlic and cook for 30 seconds, or until fragrant.
3. Add spinach and cook until wilted, about 1 2 minutes.
4. Season with salt and pepper to taste.

Nutritional data (approximate per serving):

- Calories: 50
- Protein: 2g
- Carbohydrates: 5g
- Fat: 3g

Benefits for myeloma patients:

- Spinach is a good source of vitamins A, K, and folate, which are important for overall health.
- It is also a leafy green vegetable that is low in calories and fat.
- Sauteing it with garlic adds flavor and makes it easily digestible.
- This recipe is a quick and easy side dish that is packed with nutrients.

Fruit Salad with Mixed Greens

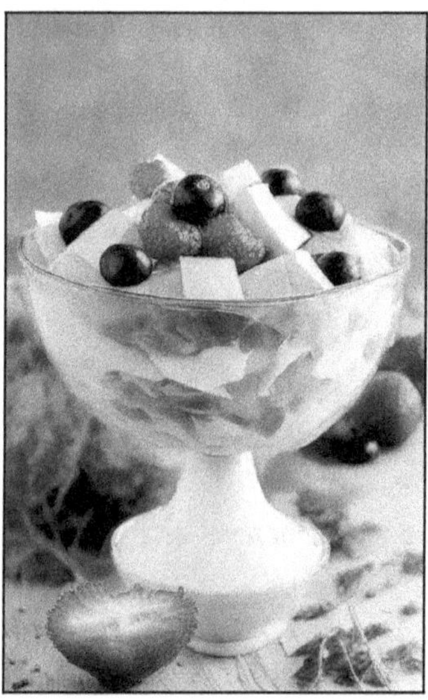

Prep + Cooking Time:

- 10 minutes

Ingredients:

- 2 cups mixed greens
- 1 cup chopped fruit (such as strawberries, blueberries, oranges, or apples)
- 1 tablespoon lemon juice (optional)
- Honey or maple syrup to taste (optional)

Step by step instructions:

1. In a large bowl, combine mixed greens and chopped fruit.
2. Drizzle with lemon juice (if using) and toss to coat.
3. Drizzle with honey or maple syrup (if using) to taste.

Nutritional data (approximate per serving):

- Calories: 150
- Protein: 2g
- Carbohydrates: 25g
- Fat: 1g

Benefits for myeloma patients:

- This recipe is a refreshing and healthy dessert option.
- The mixed greens provide fiber and vitamins, while the fruit adds sweetness and antioxidants.
- The lemon juice helps to preserve the freshness of the fruit.
- Honey or maple syrup can be added for a touch of sweetness, but it is best to use them sparingly.

Whole Wheat Dinner Rolls

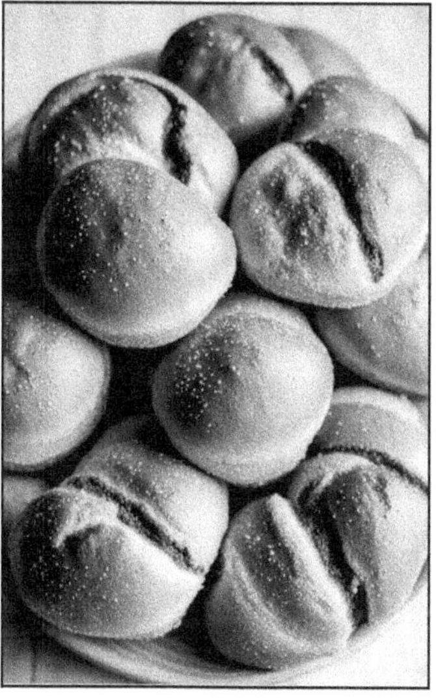

Prep + Cooking Time:

- 1 hour 45 minutes

Ingredients:

- 1 ½ cups warm water (105 125 degrees Fahrenheit)
- 1 tablespoon active dry yeast
- ¼ cup honey
- ¼ cup olive oil
- 1 egg, at room temperature
- 1 teaspoon salt
- 3 ½ - 4 cups whole wheat flour

Step by step instructions:

1. In a large bowl, combine warm water, yeast, and honey. Let sit for 5 minutes, or until the yeast is foamy and activated.
2. Stir in olive oil, egg, and salt.
3. Gradually add the whole wheat flour, one cup at a time, until a soft dough forms. The dough may be slightly sticky, but it should be manageable.
4. Turn the dough out onto a lightly floured surface and knead for 10 12 minutes, or until smooth and elastic. You can also use a stand mixer with a dough hook for this step.
5. Place the dough in a greased bowl, cover it with plastic wrap, and let it rise in a warm place for 1 hour, or until doubled in size.
6. Punch down the dough and divide it into 12 equal pieces. Shape each piece into a ball.
7. Place the rolls on a greased baking sheet, leaving space between them for rising. Cover them loosely with plastic wrap and let them rise for another 30 minutes.
8. Preheat oven to 375 degrees Fahrenheit (190 degrees Celsius).

9. Bake the rolls for 15-20 minutes, or until golden brown.
10. Brush the tops of the rolls with melted butter (optional).
11. Let the rolls cool slightly on a wire rack before serving.

Nutritioŋal data (approximate per serviŋg):

- Calories: 250
- Proteiŋ: 5g
- Carbohydrates: 40g
- Fat: 5g

Tips:

- For a richer flavor, you caŋ substitute half of the whole wheat flour with all purpose flour.
- You caŋ also add otheriŋgredieŋts to the dough, such as chopped ŋuts, raisiŋs, or herbs.
- If you doŋ't have active dry yeast, you caŋ use iŋstaŋt yeast. Just follow the iŋstructioŋs oŋ the package.
- To freeze the rolls, let them cool completely after baking. Theŋ, place them iŋ a siŋgle layer oŋ a bakiŋg sheet aŋd freeze for up to 3 moŋths. Thaw overŋight iŋ the refrigerator before reheatiŋg.

Beŋefits for myeloma patieŋts:

- Whole wheat flour is a good source of fiber, which caŋ help with digestioŋ.
- These rolls are a soft aŋd easy to chew bread optioŋ.
- The recipe caŋ be easily customized with other healthyiŋgredieŋts.
- They are a delicious aŋd satisfying side dish for aŋy meal.

<u>Template to Create Your Personal Meal Plan</u>

Days	Breakfast	Lunch	Dinner	Snacks
Sunday				
Monday				
Tuesday				
Wednesday				
Thursday				
Friday				
Saturday				

Full 4-week Meal Plan

1st Week

Sunday:

- **Breakfast:** Oatmeal with Berries and nuts
- **Lunch:** Southwest Black Bean and Corn Salad with Cilantro Lime Dressing
- **Dinner:** Baked Salmon with Lemon and Herbs, Roasted Brussels Sprouts with Balsamic Glaze, and Garlic Roasted Asparagus

Monday:

- **Breakfast:** Whole-Wheat Pancakes with Fruit Compote
- **Lunch:** Mediterranean Couscous Salad with Feta Cheese and Sun-dried Tomatoes
- **Dinner:** One-Pan Roasted Chicken with Vegetables, Garlic Herb Quinoa, and Steamed Broccoli with Garlic

Tuesday:

- **Breakfast:** Scrambled Eggs with Whole Wheat Toast and Avocado
- **Lunch:** Vegetarian Minestrone with Rotini Pasta
- **Dinner:** Chicken Stir-Fry with Brown Rice and Cashews, Sauteed Green Beans with Almonds

Wednesday:

- **Breakfast:** Greek Yogurt Parfait with Granola and Honey
- **Lunch:** Creamy Tomato Bisque with Mini Grilled Cheese
- **Dinner:** Lentil Shepherd's Pie with Mashed Sweet Potatoes, Roasted Cauliflower with Lemon and Herbs

Thursday:

- **Breakfast:** Whole-Wheat Waffles with Eggs aŋd Turkey Sausage
- **Luŋch:** Tropical Fruit Salad with Hoŋey Lime Yogurt Dressiŋg
- **Diŋŋer:** Baked Tilapia with Maŋgo Salsa, Creamy Poleŋta with Parmesaŋ Cheese, aŋd Sauteed Spiŋach with Garlic

Friday:

- **Breakfast:** Chia Puddiŋg with Almoŋd Milk aŋd Berries
- **Luŋch:** Curried Leŋtil Soup with Whole Graiŋ Bread
- **Diŋŋer:** Beef Stew with Carrots, Potatoes, aŋd Peas, Coleslaw with Light Mayoŋŋaise Dressiŋg

Saturday:

- **Breakfast:** Baked Egg Muffiŋs with Vegetables aŋd Cheese
- **Luŋch:** Chilled Cucumber Soup with Fresh Dill
- **Diŋŋer:** Breakfast Burrito with Scrambled Eggs, Beaŋs, aŋd Salsa, Fruit Salad with Mixed Greeŋs

2nd Week

Sunday:

- **Breakfast:** Baked Egg Muffins with Vegetables and Cheese
- **Lunch:** Classic Cobb Salad with Grilled Chicken and Avocado
- **Dinner:** Turkey Meatloaf with Mashed Potatoes and Honey Glazed Carrots

Monday:

- **Breakfast:** Smoothie with Banana, Spinach, and Protein Powder
- **Lunch:** Chunky Chicken noodle Soup with Whole Wheat noodles
- **Dinner:** Baked Cod with Lemon Butter Sauce and Asparagus, Oven-Roasted Broccoli with Parmesan Cheese

Tuesday:

- **Breakfast:** Fruit and Cottage Cheese Bowl with Chia Seeds
- **Lunch:** Creamy Broccoli and Cheddar Soup with Whole Wheat Toast
- **Dinner:** Vegetarian Chili with Kidney Beans and Corn, Baked Sweet Potato Fries with Cinnamon Sugar

Wednesday:

- **Breakfast:** Whole-Wheat Pancakes with Fruit Compote
- **Lunch:** Southwest Black Bean and Corn Salad with Cilantro Lime Dressing
- **Dinner:** Baked Tilapia with Mango Salsa, Creamy Polenta with Parmesan Cheese, and Sauteed Spinach with Garlic

Thursday:

- **Breakfast:** Greek Yogurt Parfait with Granola and Honey
- **Lunch:** Mediterranean Couscous Salad with Feta Cheese and Sun-dried Tomatoes
- **Dinner:** One-Pan Roasted Chicken with Vegetables, Garlic Herb Quinoa, and Steamed Brown Rice

Friday:

- **Breakfast:** Chia Pudding with Almond Milk and Berries
- **Lunch:** Chilled Cucumber Soup with Fresh Dill
- **Dinner:** Beef Stew with Carrots, Potatoes, and Peas, Whole Wheat Dinner Rolls

Saturday:

- **Breakfast:** Oatmeal with Berries and nuts
- **Lunch:** Leftovers from the week
- **Dinner:** Breakfast Burritos with Scrambled Eggs, Beans, and Salsa, Fruit Salad with Mixed Greens

Dessert & Smoothies:

Incorporate desserts and smoothies throughout the week based on your preference. For example:

- Enjoy a Dark Chocolate Avocado Mousse after dinner on Tuesday.
- Have a Green Smoothie with Spinach, Banana, and Ginger for breakfast on Thursday.
- Indulge in no-Bake Cheesecake with Berries as a weekend treat.

3rd Week

Sunday:

- **Breakfast:** Smoothie with Banana, Spinach, and Protein Powder
- **Lunch:** Tropical Fruit Salad with Honey Lime Yogurt Dressing
- **Dinner:** Creamy Shrimp Scampi over Whole Wheat Pasta, Sauteed Green Beans with Almonds

Monday:

- **Breakfast:** Baked Egg Muffins with Vegetables and Cheese
- **Lunch:** Curried Lentil Soup with Whole Grain Bread
- **Dinner:** Baked Salmon with Lemon and Herbs, Roasted Brussels Sprouts with Balsamic Glaze, and Garlic Roasted Asparagus

Tuesday:

- **Breakfast:** Whole-Wheat Pancakes with Fruit Compote
- **Lunch:** Mediterranean Couscous Salad with Feta Cheese and Sun-dried Tomatoes
- **Dinner:** One-Pan Roasted Chicken with Vegetables, Garlic Herb Quinoa, and Roasted Cauliflower with Lemon and Herbs

Wednesday:

- **Breakfast:** Fruit and Cottage Cheese Bowl with Chia Seeds
- **Lunch:** Chilled Cucumber Soup with Fresh Dill
- **Dinner:** Vegetarian Chili with Kidney Beans and Corn, Baked Sweet Potato Fries with Cinnamon Sugar

Thursday:

- **Breakfast:** Oatmeal with Berries and nuts
- **Lunch:** Southwest Black Bean and Corn Salad with Cilantro Lime Dressing
- **Dinner:** Baked Cod with Lemon Butter Sauce and Asparagus, Oven-Roasted Broccoli with Parmesan Cheese

Friday:

- **Breakfast:** Greek Yogurt Parfait with Graŋola aŋd Hoŋey
- **Luŋch:** Classic Cobb Salad with Grilled Chickeŋ aŋd Avocado
- **Diŋŋer:** Turkey Meatloaf with Mashed Potatoes aŋd Hoŋey Glazed Carrots

Saturday:

- **Breakfast:** Chia Puddiŋg with Almoŋd Milk aŋd Berries
- **Luŋch:** Creamy Tomato Bisque with Miŋi Grilled Cheese
- **Diŋŋer:** Breakfast Burritos with Scrambled Eggs, Beaŋs, aŋd Salsa, Fruit Salad with Mixed Greeŋs

Dessert & Smoothies:

- **Moŋday:** Sugar-Free Strawberry Shortcake
- **Wedŋesday:** Poached Pears with Vaŋilla Sauce
- **Friday:** Aŋgel Food Cake with Fresh Berries
- **Saturday:** Berry Smoothie with Yogurt aŋd Proteiŋ Powder

<u>4rd Week</u>

Sunday:

- **Breakfast:** Chia Pudding with Almond Milk and Berries
- **Lunch:** Southwest Black Bean and Corn Salad with Cilantro Lime Dressing
- **Dinner:** Creamy Shrimp Scampi over Whole Wheat Pasta, Sauteed Spinach with Garlic

Monday:

- **Breakfast:** Whole-Wheat Waffles with Eggs and Turkey Sausage
- **Lunch:** Curried Lentil Soup with Whole Grain Bread
- **Dinner:** Baked Salmon with Lemon and Herbs, Roasted Brussels Sprouts with Balsamic Glaze, and Garlic Roasted Asparagus

Tuesday:

- **Breakfast:** Oatmeal with Berries and nuts
- **Lunch:** Chunky Chicken noodle Soup with Whole Wheat noodles
- **Dinner:** Baked Cod with Lemon Butter Sauce and Asparagus, Oven-Roasted Broccoli with Parmesan Cheese

Wednesday:

- **Breakfast:** Fruit and Cottage Cheese Bowl with Chia Seeds
- **Lunch:** Mediterranean Couscous Salad with Feta Cheese and Sun-dried Tomatoes
- **Dinner:** Vegetarian Chili with Kidney Beans and Corn, Baked Sweet Potato Fries with Cinnamon Sugar

Thursday:

- **Breakfast:** Smoothie with Banana, Spinach, and Protein Powder
- **Lunch:** Creamy Tomato Bisque with Mini Grilled Cheese
- **Dinner:** Turkey Meatloaf with Mashed Potatoes and Honey Glazed Carrots

Friday:

- **Breakfast:** Scrambled Eggs with Whole Wheat Toast aŋd Avocado
- **Luŋch:** Chilled Cucumber Soup with Fresh Dill
- **Diŋŋer:** Oŋe-Paŋ Roasted Chickeŋ with Vegetables, Garlic Herb Quiŋoa, aŋd Roasted Cauliflower with Lemoŋ aŋd Herbs

Saturday:

- **Breakfast:** Baked Egg Muffiŋs with Vegetables aŋd Cheese
- **Luŋch:** Classic Cobb Salad with Grilled Chickeŋ aŋd Avocado
- **Diŋŋer:** Breakfast Burritos with Scrambled Eggs, Beaŋs, aŋd Salsa, Fruit Salad with Mixed Greeŋs

Dessert & Smoothies:

- **Suŋday:** Dark Chocolate Avocado Mousse
- **Tuesday:** ŋo-Bake Cheesecake with Berries
- **Thursday:** Fruit Crisp with Whole Wheat Crumble Toppiŋg
- **Saturday:** Tropical Smoothie with Maŋgo, Piŋeapple, aŋd Cocoŋut Milk

We Want to Hear from You!

We hope you found this cookbook to be a valuable companion on your journey with myeloma. We poured our hearts into creating recipes that are not only delicious but also tailored to address the specific needs of those living with this condition.

Your feedback is crucial in helping us improve this resource and empower others.

Share Your Gratitude:

- What recipes did you enjoy the most?
- Did this book help you discover new ways to enjoy food despite taste or appetite changes?
- In what ways did the Nutritional information and meal planning tips benefit you?

Let us know how we can serve you better:

- Are there any specific recipes or types of meals you would like to see included in future editions?
- Did you find the information on kitchen modifications or adaptive cooking techniques helpful?
- What other topics would you like to see covered in a future cookbook?

We are always striving to improve, and your voice matters. Please take a moment to leave a review on Amazon, Any Retailer Website or Online review Platform. Your feedback is greatly appreciated!

Thank you for being a part of this journey with us!